TECHNICAL REPORT

Achieving Strong Teamwork Practices in Hospital Labor and Delivery Units

Donna O. Farley, Melony E. Sorbero,
Susan L. Lovejoy, Mary Salisbury

Prepared for the Office of the Secretary of Defense

Center for Military Health Policy Research

A JOINT ENDEAVOR OF RAND HEALTH AND THE
RAND NATIONAL DEFENSE RESEARCH INSTITUTE

The research reported here was sponsored by the Office of the Secretary of Defense (OSD). The research was conducted jointly by the Center for Military Health Policy Research, a RAND Health program, and the Forces and Resources Policy Center, a RAND National Defense Research Institute (NDRI) program. NDRI is a federally funded research and development center sponsored by the OSD, the Joint Staff, the Unified Combatant Commands, the Navy, the Marine Corps, the defense agencies, and the defense Intelligence Community under Contract W74V8H-06-C-0002.

Library of Congress Control Number: 2010938595

ISBN: 978-0-8330-5055-7

The RAND Corporation is a nonprofit institution that helps improve policy and decisionmaking through research and analysis. RAND's publications do not necessarily reflect the opinions of its research clients and sponsors.

RAND® is a registered trademark.

Published 2010 by the RAND Corporation
1776 Main Street, P.O. Box 2138, Santa Monica, CA 90407-2138
1200 South Hayes Street, Arlington, VA 22202-5050
4570 Fifth Avenue, Suite 600, Pittsburgh, PA 15213-2665
RAND URL: http://www.rand.org/
To order RAND documents or to obtain additional information, contact
Distribution Services: Telephone: (310) 451-7002;
Fax: (310) 451-6915; Email: order@rand.org

Preface

The U.S. Department of Defense (DoD) Patient Safety Program Office of the TRICARE Management Activity (TMA) provides training and support for the health-care facilities operated by military services to help strengthen their use of effective teamwork practices. In 2002, TMA funded a study aimed to assess the effects of teamwork training for labor and delivery teams on patient safety and other outcomes for mothers and newborns (Nielsen et al., 2007). The study presented in this report is a successor to the 2002 study, with the goal of addressing a number of the issues raised from the earlier study's findings. Using a case-study design, this study has focused on learning from the experiences of five labor and delivery units in implementing teamwork practices for the staff working in their units. Through a combination of process and outcome assessments, using site visits, interviews, staff surveys, and analysis of patient outcomes, the study sought to understand what is required for health-care organizations to achieve effective and sustainable teamwork practices.

The contents of this report will be of interest to national and state policymakers, health-care organizations, health researchers, and others involved in efforts to improve teamwork practices in health-care organizations.

This research was sponsored by Patient Safety Program Office of the Assistant Secretary of Defense/Health Affairs TRICARE Management Activity and conducted jointly by RAND Health's Center for Military Health Policy Research and the Forces and Resources Policy Center of the RAND National Defense Research Institute (NDRI). The Center for Military Health Policy Research taps RAND expertise in both defense and health policy to conduct research for the Department of Defense, the Veterans Administration, and non-profit organizations. RAND Health aims to transform the well-being of all people by solving complex problems in health and health care. NDRI is a federally funded research and development center sponsored by the Office of the Secretary of Defense, the Joint Staff, the Unified Combatant Commands, the Navy, the Marine Corps, the defense agencies, and the defense Intelligence Community.

For more information on the Center for Military Health Policy Research, see http://www.rand.org/multi/military/ or contact the co-Directors (contact information is provided on the web page). For more information on the Forces and Resources Policy Center, see http://www.rand.org/nsrd/about/frp.html or contact the Director (contact information is provided on the web page).

Contents

Figures

Tables

Summary

This study of teamwork-improvement initiatives in hospital labor and delivery (L&D) units was designed to document and learn from the experiences and outcomes of five L&D units as they implemented improvements in their teamwork practices over a one-year period. The study had the following objectives:

- *Objective 1:* Better understand the conditions and actions required for hospital L&D units to achieve effective and sustainable teamwork practices.
- *Objective 2:* Assess the extent to which successful adoption of teamwork practices may influence the experiences of L&D staff and patient outcomes.

Background

Inadequate teamwork and communication during health-care delivery contributes to adverse patient events (Petersen et al., 1994; Kachalia et al., 2007; Arora et al., 2007). Teamwork is a sustained effort using shared skills (Morey, Simon, Jay, Wears, et al., 2002). Installing a team structure in an organization, however, does not automatically result in effective teamwork. Effective team performance requires cooperation among team members in pursuing a shared goal, effective communications within the team, adequate organizational resources and support, and shared acknowledgement of participating members' roles and abilities (McGrath, 1984; Campion, Medsker, and Higgs, 1993; Stevens and Campion, 1994).

MedTeams™ and TeamSTEPPS are two generations of a health-care teamwork model based on crew resource management (CRM) (Morey, Simon, Jay, and Rice, 2002; Morey, Simon, Jay, Wears, et al., 2002). The two models are similar, with TeamSTEPPS being a more-recent refinement of the MedTeams model. Both are evidence-based systems to improve teamwork among health-care professionals. These models consist of four teamwork competency sets, along with a set of specific teamwork skills or practices (to which we refer as *practices* in this report). The four competency sets (DoD, 2005) are as follows:

- *leadership:* the ability to direct and coordinate the activities of other team members
- *situation monitoring:* the process of actively scanning situational elements to gain awareness of the situation in which the team functions
- *mutual support:* the ability to anticipate and support other team members' needs through accurate knowledge about their responsibilities and workload
- *communication:* the process by which information is clearly and accurately exchanged among team members.

Study Approach and Design

Basic Study Design

The study design was based on a quality improvement (QI) framework. According to the QI model, effective quality improvement comes about through regular, incremental changes in the practices of interest, guided by measurement, monitoring, and feedback on performance. A successful QI initiative will motivate staff to plan, execute, and evaluate organizational change (Imai, 1986; Solberg et al., 1998; Cox, Wilcock, and Young, 1999; Glezerman et al., 1999; Schwab et al., 1999; Gandhi et al., 2000; Harris et al., 2000; Laurila et al., 2001).

The use of the QI framework and a case-study approach allowed us to take advantage of the natural variation in implementation activities across five participating L&D sites. The ultimate goal was for all the L&D units to fully implement all the practices in the teamwork model, regardless of which model (MedTeams or TeamSTEPPS) they chose. Each unit developed and carried out an implementation strategy that it felt worked best for its unit and team and reflected its situation and performance issues. This approach acknowledges that each organization has unique circumstances and needs and, therefore, will be most effective by pursuing a QI strategy that responds to its unique situation.

The study design included a process evaluation, through which we explored, as case studies, the multiple factors involved in the implementation processes of the five participating L&D units. The longitudinal design for the process evaluation enabled us to observe the L&D units for a year and to gain an understanding of (1) changes in the experiences of the L&D units in implementing teamwork-practice improvements and (2) the evolution of their implementation activities over time in response to those experiences. The design also included an outcome evaluation, in which we used a before-and-after design for analysis of effects on staff perceptions and knowledge and a time-series design for analysis of effects on patient outcomes.

Participating Labor and Delivery Units

Five hospitals participated in this study: two military and three civilian hospitals. We selected these L&D units for participation because they had made an explicit commitment to improving teamwork practices.

- *Site 1:* This site is a large L&D unit in a community hospital with no medical residency program. The unit had not acted to implement teamwork improvements until the start of this study. When work began, it was with a strong sense of urgency because the hospital board of directors had made teamwork a high priority and was pushing for fast action. Its basic approach was structured and strongly proactive.
- *Site 2:* This site is an academic medical center in an urban area and is a referral center for other hospitals (many of them difficult-delivery cases). The unit had begun teamwork improvement in the year before this study started, but its momentum had eroded. It used this study to inject new energy into the work to further its progress. The L&D unit took an approach of pursuing incremental progress by implementing subsets of teamwork practices over time, rather than working with many practices at once.
- *Site 3:* This site is a large L&D unit in a suburban hospital with a medical residency program. Although it had been an intervention site in the original L&D teamwork study, the site had not previously implemented most aspects of teamwork practices. Its approach was to work on a variety of specific practices using a flexible strategy.

- *Site 4:* This site is a large L&D unit in a regional referral center with a medical residency program. It had been an intervention site in the original L&D teamwork study, and it had already implemented many aspects of teamwork practices. As a result, it took a gradual, incremental approach to working with specific teamwork practices during the study, focusing on refining and reinforcing individual practices.
- *Site 5:* This site also is a large L&D unit in a regional referral center with a medical residency program. The unit had not acted to implement teamwork improvements until the start of this study. It took an incremental approach to working with specific teamwork practices, taking time to reinforce those being implemented at each time.

The participating hospitals applied two basic strategies for implementing improved teamwork practices: (1) training for staff in the skills and practices involved in team-based care and (2) carrying out a variety of actions to encourage L&D staff to adopt teamwork practices as part of their care processes.

Research Questions for the Study

The evaluation was designed to address its two objectives and four associated research questions, two of which addressed each study objective, as summarized in this section. The first objective was addressed by the process evaluation, and the second objective by the outcome evaluation.

- *Objective 1:* Better understand the conditions and actions required for hospital L&D units to achieve effective and sustainable teamwork practices, by asking the following research questions:
  - What training and actions are required to achieve a high level of teamwork in the L&D process?
  - How strongly do self-reported experiences in implementing teamwork improvements correlate with actual levels of teamwork as measured by direct observation of the L&D process? (Note that, in order to examine the extent to which the sites had strengthened their teamwork practices, we used a combination of qualitative, self-reported interview data and observation data. Because we did not have baseline observation data [due to budget constraints], we could not directly examine changes in observed practices from baseline to the end of the study.)
- *Objective 2.* Assess the extent to which successful adoption of teamwork practices may influence staff experiences and patient outcomes, by asking the following research questions:
  - How does achieving effective teamwork affect the perceptions and experiences of staff working in L&D units?
  - What effects does effective teamwork have on L&D outcomes for mothers and newborn infants?

The logic model in Figure S.1 identifies the steps taken by the hospitals in implementing teamwork improvements and shows how the evaluation interfaced with those activities. The middle row of the model ("Hospital L&D units") represents a three-step sequence of teamwork status, starting with baseline status, moving to changes in teamwork practices resulting from improvement activities, and ultimately leading to improved team-based care. The top row of

Figure S.1
Evaluation Components for the Labor and Delivery Teamwork Training Study

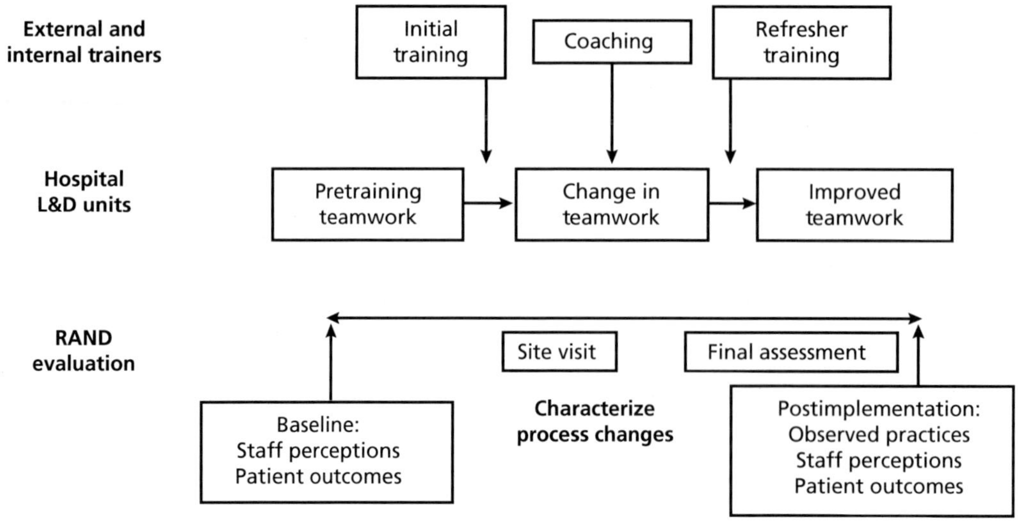

RAND *TR842-S.1*

the model represents the training provided, including the initial training of unit staff, follow-up coaching, and refresher training over time. Finally, the bottom row of the model represents the approach and data-collection schedule for our evaluation of the implementation process.

Data Collection

Process Evaluation. We collected data for the process evaluation to document the evolution of the L&D units' teamwork-improvement activities, successes achieved, challenges encountered, and the pace at which they adopted the specific teamwork practices delineated in either the MedTeams or TeamSTEPPS curriculum. We gathered data on the extent to which they implemented teamwork training, took advantage of coaching, initiated other initiatives, or experienced disruptions that might affect process and outcome measures.

Outcome Evaluation. Data for measuring changes in staff perceptions and knowledge over time were collected in a staff survey conducted twice during the study period. To estimate effects on patients, we used the Adverse Outcome Index (AOI) and the Weighted Adverse Outcome Score (WAOS), which are L&D outcome measures developed as part of the previous L&D clinical trial funded by DoD (Mann et al., 2006). The AOI is a measure of the frequency of adverse delivery outcomes divided by the total number of deliveries. The WAOS captures the severity of these outcomes by weighting each outcome measure by a weight that represents the severity of the outcome. The National Perinatal Information Center (NPIC) calculated hospital-level rates for these measures on a quarterly basis, using hospital discharge data provided to it by the participating hospitals.

Findings: Teamwork Implementation

The results of the process evaluation highlighted that, whereas the L&D units used a diversity of implementation approaches, several key factors appear to be required for achieving teamwork improvements. Here, we summarize our results for each of the research questions addressed by the process evaluation.

What Training and Actions Are Required to Achieve a High Level of Teamwork in the Labor and Delivery Process?

The key factors required for successful implementation appear to be early emphasis on the teamwork competency of communication, along with effective training and coaching, support of a facilitator to keep the process on track, and perseverance in working toward practice adoption by staff working on the unit. The other three teamwork competencies—leadership, situation awareness, and mutual support—also are important to achieve, and they were addressed successfully using a variety of approaches. For choices regarding introduction of the specific teamwork practices, the team huddle/brief (a tool for reinforcing the plans already in place for the treatment of patients, assessing the need to change plans, and developing a shared understanding of the plan of care among team members) is an important practice to adopt early in the implementation process. It appears that the remaining practices can be addressed in the order that each unit finds to be most appropriate. (See Appendix A for a complete list and definitions of the specific team practices.)

The sites came to recognize the importance of providing initial teamwork training for all staff. Several of the sites did initial training for only part of their staff because of budget constraints or operational trade-offs. All of these sites stated that this led to slower staff buy-in and delays in adoption of practices. The sites also reported substantial difficulties in getting staff trained later using coaching or informal training.

Typical challenges the sites experienced from external sources included staff shortages, construction projects, and competing initiatives. A common internal challenge was initial staff resistance to teamwork improvement. Such resistance tended to decline with time as staff gained experience with teamwork and saw its benefits. Tension between physicians and nurses can also be expected early in the implementation process.

How Strongly Do Self-Reported Experiences in Implementing Teamwork Improvements Correlate with Actual Levels of Teamwork as Measured by Direct Observation of the Labor and Delivery Process?

The observation scores for teamwork performance varied across sites, across time periods within sites, and across teamwork aspects within sites. The levels and variations in teamwork scores for each site were consistent with self-reported implementation status as of the end of the study. These results highlight the potential value of using observational studies to track progress as teams try to improve teamwork practices. Observations by an external expert can provide objective data to identify issues and guide subsequent implementation actions.

Findings: Effects of Teamwork Improvement on Staff and Patients

The outcome-evaluation results suggested that the teamwork implementation efforts of the participating L&D units influenced staff experiences working in the units, but effects for maternal and newborn outcomes were observable only for site 2. We summarize here what we learned regarding each of the research questions addressed by the outcome evaluation.

How Does Achieving Effective Teamwork Affect the Perceptions and Experiences of Staff Working in Labor and Delivery Units?

We found improvements in staff perceptions of teamwork, especially for domains closest to teamwork in the L&D units—teamwork practices, communication openness, and teamwork climate—as well as for quality of work-life and teamwork knowledge. However, the sites varied with respect to the domains for which staff perceptions improved, ranging from improvements for all five domains for site 1 to improvement in only one domain for site 3.

We also found significant relationships between improvements in L&D unit staff perceptions and two of the three measures for implementation actions identified as potentially important—coaching and extent of initial training and facilitator support during the teamwork implementation process. Their effects varied across the domains of staff perceptions. Staff perceptions did not appear to be affected by how many of the specific teamwork practices the units had actually implemented. These results suggest that successful adoption of a large number of the specific teamwork practices may not be an important factor in changing staff perceptions and knowledge of teamwork in the L&D units.

What Effects Does Effective Teamwork Have on Labor and Delivery Outcomes for Mothers and Newborn Infants?

The only effect found for maternal and newborn outcomes was a reduction in the AOI for site 2 during the teamwork implementation period. Although the AOI trend for site 2 declined, its WAOS trend did not change, nor were there changes in WAOS trends for the other sites. These results suggest that site 2 might have reduced the frequency of less-severe patient events but not total overall severity. This interpretation was supported by the site lead, who reported that the team continued to experience infrequent, high-severity events, even though overall event frequency had declined.

These generally null findings may reflect the nature of the outcome measures used. Most of them are very low-frequency adverse events, for which stable trends are difficult to establish. The successes reported by the participating L&D units during the study suggested that their work was having effects on their care delivery for patients, which pointed to other possible candidate measures. For example, sites reported that they affected emergency Cesarean sections (C-sections), C-section infection rates, and customer satisfaction.

Synthesis of Findings

This longitudinal study provided rich information about the processes and dynamics of improving teamwork practices. The study also revealed the complexities of these processes, which require a major cultural change within the L&D units and cannot be done quickly. To assess the relationships between the L&D units' implementation processes and their associated outcomes, we combined the results from the process evaluation and outcome evaluation. In Table S.1, we delineate the implementation methods used by each L&D unit, characterize the unit's progress in adopting teamwork practices, and list effects on outcomes. We group the sites according to whether they had pursued teamwork improvements before the study began.

The experiences of these L&D units indicate that substantial progress is possible in one year of implementing teamwork practices and that proximal outcomes, such as staff knowledge and perceptions, can be improved. More than a year of implementation effort is required

Table S.1
Summary of Results Regarding Implementation Progress and Outcome Changes, by Site

Progress	No Previous Work on Teamwork			Previously Worked on Teamwork	
	Site 1	Site 3	Site 5	Site 2	Site 4
Baseline status	No work	No work	No work	Work	Work
Implementation action					
Proactive strategy[a]	xxx	x	xx	xx	x
Active implementation team[a]	xxx	xx	xx	xx	x
Had a facilitator	x			x	
Trained all staff	x			x	
Used ongoing coaching	x	x		x	
Practices implemented[b]	8	3	3	4	3
Observed teamwork practices[c]	3.3–4.0	2.8–3.0	3.4–3.9	3.7–4.1	4.5–4.6
Outcome changes					
Staff perceptions improved	5	1	4	3	3
Reduction in AOI				x	

[a] x = weak. xx = moderate. xxx = strong.

[b] Of a total of nine teamwork practices.

[c] Observed at the end of the study; average scores out of a total of 5 points.

to achieve a high level of performance on teamwork practices. At the end of the study, all of the sites reported that their work was not done and that they intended to continue working on teamwork improvements. The scores the five sites received in the observation study support this premise. The two sites that had worked on teamwork prior to the study had higher scores than the other three sites.

These results suggest that two dynamics might be involved in later years of implementation. First, momentum from the first year might continue into later years, such that subsequent implementation might reinforce continued improvement. This premise is supported by the high performance scores of sites 2 and 4. Second, it might not be possible to sustain high intensity in implementation beyond the first year. Thus, the less-intense strategies of these two sites might represent expected levels of activity for later implementation years.

Implications

The study results reinforce the importance of developing and implementing a well-crafted strategy by training staff in the L&D units, working with staff to introduce practices, and providing coaching on effective use of those practices. We see this in the summary of results from the process evaluation. We also hear these messages in the retrospective assessments by the participating L&D units, including the importance of persevering in the pursuit of their strategy over time (summarized in Chapter Three). These findings are consistent with the guidance provided by the Agency for Healthcare Research and Quality (AHRQ) on its TeamSTEPPS website (AHRQ, undated).

The study identified some key factors required by any given strategy for teamwork improvement, but it did not point to a standard template for implementation. This result implies that there may not be one fixed "intervention" that could be tested in comparative-control studies to develop further evidence for teamwork practices.

We selected L&D units for the study that had committed to achieving teamwork improvement. We made this selection based on published evidence that successful adoption of new practices requires hard work and perseverance. This premise was supported by the insights obtained from the participating L&D units, all of which highlighted the need for such commitment to make progress. Therefore, we identify the reference group for generalizability as being other L&D units that also are committed to making such improvements. It is possible that, if other L&D units were observed as additional case studies, different factors or strategies might emerge that also influence implementation success. We encourage further work in this area to test these findings with additional case studies, which could help build a depth of evidence across a larger number of organizations.

Acknowledgments

We gratefully acknowledge the participation of the numerous leaders and staff working in the five L&D units that we tracked and studied for longer than a year. Their commitment to the teamwork improvements they were implementing, as well as to this research, created a constructive environment that allowed us to learn from them and provide feedback as their implementation activities moved forward. They were candid and thoughtful in the information they provided, which yielded a rich information base for our analyses.

We also thank our DoD project officer, Heidi King, Patient Safety Program Office, TRICARE Management Activity, who has continued to be an active guide and supporter of our work and has provided valuable insights on the realities of teamwork implementation from her experience working with numerous military hospitals. We also thank Deidre Gifford and, at RAND, John Adams for their helpful comments on an earlier draft of this report. Any errors of fact or interpretation in this report remain the responsibility of the authors.

Abbreviations

AHRQ	Agency for Healthcare Research and Quality
AOI	Adverse Outcome Index
BARS	behaviorally anchored rating scale
BIDMC	Beth Israel Deaconess Medical Center
CAHPS	Consumer Assessment of Healthcare Providers and Systems
C-section	Cesarean section
CRM	crew resource management
DESC	describe, express, suggest, and consequences
DoD	U.S. Department of Defense
HSOPS	Hospital Survey on Patient Safety Culture
ICU	intensive-care unit
I'M SAFE	illness, medication, stress, alcohol/drugs, fatigue, eating, elimination, and emotions
IOM	Institute of Medicine
IRB	institutional review board
L&D	labor and delivery
MD	medical doctor
NICU	neonatal intensive-care unit
NPIC	National Perinatal Information Center
OB	obstetrics
OR	operating room
PSC	patient service coordinator
QI	quality improvement

Qx	quarter x, where x = the number of quarters since implementation began (e.g., implementation begins in Q1)
RN	registered nurse
SAQ	Safety Attitude Questionnaire
SBAR	situation, background, assessment, and recommendation
SI	severity index
STEP	status of patient, team members, environment, and progress
SWAT	strength, weakness, and threat analysis
TMA	TRICARE Management Activity
TPAC	teamwork-practice award card
WAOS	Weighted Adverse Outcome Score

CHAPTER ONE

Introduction and Background

Research Objectives

This study was designed to document and learn from the experiences and outcomes of five hospital labor and delivery (L&D) units as they implemented improvements in their teamwork practices over a one-year period. The study had the following objectives:

- *Objective 1:* Better understand the conditions and actions required for hospital L&D units to achieve effective and sustainable teamwork practices.
- *Objective 2:* Assess the extent to which successful adoption of teamwork practices may influence the experiences of staff working in the units and outcomes for patients.

It is well documented in the quality-improvement (QI) literature that successful implementation of new or improved health-care practices requires commitment and perseverance by the providers carrying out the implementation, coupled with well-designed intervention strategies (Kuperman et al., 1991; Messina, 1997; Larson, 2002; Lindenauer et al., 2004; Pronovost and Holzmueller, 2004). It also is understood that many patient-safety practices are system-level interventions that involve multiple actions functioning collectively to achieve effective practice adoption (Leape, Brennan, et al., 1991; Leape, Berwick, and Bates, 2002; Farley et al., 2007, Chapter Four).

Teamwork practices, also referred to as *team-based care*, represent one system-level patient-safety practice. Using a system theory model, team-based care encompasses team inputs, team processes, and team outputs, all of which occur over time. Team inputs include the characteristics of the tasks to be performed, the elements of the context in which work occurs, and the attitudes that its members bring to a situation involving teamwork. Team processes are team interactions and coordination necessary to achieve specific goals. Team outputs consist of products derived from the team's collective efforts (McGrath, 1984; Hackman, 1987; Ilgen, 1999).

To meet our research objectives, we designed this study to address both the multifaceted nature of team-based care and the known requirements for successful implementation. We sought to examine the underlying relationships between teamwork training provided to staff in the L&D units and the subsequent actions that the L&D units implemented to improve their teamwork practices (with the goal of achieving strong, team-based care). We specifically wanted to understand which aspects of the implementation strategies and actions appeared to be most important to achieve successful adoption of the teamwork practices, and to assess effects of those practices on relevant outcomes.

Background

The Value of Teamwork in Health-Care Delivery

Inadequate teamwork and communication during provision of health-care services have been identified as important factors in adverse events that occur for patients. For example, many adverse events are related to communication failures and errors in patient hand-offs (e.g., from one department to another during an inpatient stay, or from one provider to another in ambulatory care), which could be prevented by use of effective teamwork practices, including structured communication methods (Petersen et al., 1994; Kachalia et al., 2007; Arora et al., 2007).

Recognizing the importance of teamwork and communication in medical care and patient safety, and their omission from medical training, the Institute of Medicine (IOM) noted in its report *To Err Is Human: Building a Safer Health System* (Kohn, Corrigan, and Donaldson, 2000) that approaches to developing effective teams were an area needing the attention of the Agency for Healthcare Research and Quality (AHRQ) and private foundations. The IOM has also recommended establishing patient-safety programs that provide "interdisciplinary team training programs for providers that incorporate proven methods of team training, such as simulation."

Teamwork is a sustained effort performed using a shared set of teamwork skills, although it does not require team members to work together permanently (Morey, Simon, Jay, Wears, et al., 2002). Installation of a team structure in an organization, however, does not automatically result in effective teamwork. Effective team performance requires that team members be willing to cooperate in pursuing a shared goal, such as patient safety. Effective teamwork also depends on effective communications within the team, adequate organizational resources and support, and shared acknowledgement of each participating member's roles and abilities (McGrath, 1984; Campion, Medsker, and Higgs, 1993; Stevens and Campion, 1994).

Although numerous models of effective teamwork exist, recent models focus on the specific competencies that individual team members need to possess to engage successfully in teamwork (Cannon-Bowers et al., 1995). Three types of competencies have been identified as being critical for effective teamwork: (1) teamwork-related knowledge, (2) teamwork-related skills, and (3) teamwork-related attitudes (Cannon-Bowers et al., 1995; Stevens and Campion, 1994; O'Neil, Chung, and Brown, 1997).

An important reference point for health-care teamwork models has been the crew resource management (CRM) concept that has been widely used in aviation to improve flight safety. CRM is a training model that emphasizes the role of human factors in high-risk, high-stress environments, which can apply to many health-care situations. The scientific evidence for application of CRM teamwork principles to medicine was examined in the patient-safety evidence report *Making Health Care Safer: A Critical Analysis of Patient Safety Practices* (AHRQ, 2001), which evaluated current evidence regarding the effectiveness of a total of 79 patient-safety practices.

The evidence report rated the evidence for teamwork practices as being at a level of lower impact or strength of evidence (the other three rating categories were highest, medium, or lowest impact or strength of evidence). It found that, as of 2001, most studies of CRM and other teamwork practices focused on the quality of teamwork training and that no evidence was available yet that linked improvements in team performance to better safety outcomes. The report also indicated that further research on teamwork practices was likely to be beneficial (the other category was likely to be highly beneficial) (AHRQ, 2001). Subsequent research has generated additional findings that address teamwork practices, although evidence regarding teamwork's effects on improvements in patient-safety outcomes continues to be limited (Sorbero et al., 2008).

The National Quality Forum has identified team-based care as one of 30 practices included in its list of safe practices, which was first established in 2003 and has been updated twice since then (NQF, 2003, 2007, 2009), thus making such care a priority for implementation by U.S. health-care providers. In addition, AHRQ has developed a toolkit to support providers in implementing TeamSTEPPS, a model of teamwork originally developed by the U.S. Department of Defense (DoD) that has been used by hospitals across the United States (AHRQ, undated; Morey, Simon, Jay, and Rice, 2002; Morey, Simon, Jay, Wears, et al., 2002).

The MedTeams and TeamSTEPPS Systems

MedTeams and TeamSTEPPS are two generations of a health-care teamwork model developed based on CRM principles (Morey, Simon, Jay, and Rice, 2002; Morey, Simon, Jay, Wears, et al., 2002). The two models are closely similar, with TeamSTEPPS being a more-recent refinement of the MedTeams model. MedTeams/TeamSTEPPS is an evidence-based teamwork system to improve communication and teamwork skills among health-care professionals. Some of the L&D units participating in this study worked with the MedTeams model, which was in use at the time they first became involved in teamwork improvement, and others worked with the more-recent TeamSTEPPS model. The training provided to all the L&D units at the start of this study used the TeamSTEPPS model.

The model contents consist of a set of basic teamwork competency sets that should be in place in an organization, along with a set of specific teamwork practices through which the teamwork competencies can be achieved. The models are compared in Table 1.1, organized according to a set of criteria for effective teamwork training (Salas, Rhodenizer, and Bowers, 2000). The two models are similar, with only minor differences seen in their sets of key competencies and the specific teamwork practices.

We organized our data collection for the evaluation based on the TeamSTEPPS competencies and teamwork practices. The four basic competency sets of teamwork specified in TeamSTEPPS are defined as follows (DoD, 2005):

- *leadership:* the ability to direct and coordinate the activities of other team members
- *situation monitoring:* the process of actively scanning situational elements to gain awareness of the situation in which the team functions
- *mutual support:* the ability to anticipate and support other team members' needs through accurate knowledge about their responsibilities and workload
- *communication:* the process by which information is clearly and accurately exchanged among team members.

The teamwork practices to be applied to achieve successful performance in the four teamwork competencies are as follows (DoD, 2005):

- team huddle/brief
- status of patient, team members, environment, and progress (STEP)
- debriefs
- the two-challenge rule

Table 1.1

Comparison of TeamSTEPPS and MedTeams, Organized by Criteria for Assessing Teamwork Training Programs

Training Criterion	TeamSTEPPS	MedTeams
Behavior-based curriculum	4- to 5-hour training	6-hour training
Provides tools and approaches for measuring teamwork	Patient and staff satisfaction AHRQ surveys on patient-safety culture	Patient and staff satisfaction Team behavior observations
Utilizes scenario-based training	Real-case vignettes Videotaped vignettes	Real-case vignettes
Evaluates training	Course evaluation	Course evaluation
Instills principles of practice and feedback	Real-case vignettes Practical application activities Scenario-based role play and coaching practicum	Real-case vignettes Test-your-knowledge activities Scenario-based role play and coaching practicum
Utilizes an enterprise view of training effectiveness	Training and evaluation performed locally but monitored and managed centrally	Training and evaluation performed locally but monitored and managed centrally
Instills principles of teams and teamwork	Train-the-trainer model, CRM-based	Train-the-trainer model, 11 CRM-based
	Key competencies: leadership, situation monitoring, mutual support, communication	Key competencies: team structure and formation, planning and problem-solving, communication, workload management, improve team skills
	Teamwork practices: team huddle/brief, debriefs, STEP, two-challenge rule, DESC script, collaboration, SBAR, call-outs, check-backs, hand-off techniques	Teamwork practices: team structure and meeting, situation awareness, shared mental model, cross-monitoring, two-challenge rule, check-back, task assistance, teamwork review, situational teaching and learning, peer coaching

- describe, express, suggest, and consequences (DESC) script
- collaboration
- situation, background, assessment, and recommendation (SBAR)
- call-outs
- check-backs
- hand-off techniques.

Each of the practices is mapped to one of the four basic teamwork competencies, thus providing an implementation structure for health-care providers. These specific teamwork practices are described in Appendix A.

A Clinical Trial That Tested Teamwork Practices

The need for additional evidence regarding the effectiveness of team-based care was addressed in a cluster-randomized control trial conducted from 2002 through 2004. This study assessed the effects of teamwork training for L&D teams on patient safety and other outcomes for mothers and their newly delivered infants (Nielsen et al., 2007).

That study was performed to validate the MedTeams teamwork training system in the L&D setting. DoD, Beth Israel Deaconess Medical Center (BIDMC), and Controlled Risk Insurance Company/Risk Management Foundation (CRICO/RMF) funded the study. L&D units in 15 civilian and military hospitals participated in the study, with the units being randomly assigned to intervention and control groups. L&D staff in the intervention group were trained using a standardized teamwork-training curriculum based on CRM that emphasized communication and team structure. Those in the control group did not receive this training.

This training intervention did not have a detectable effect on the patient outcomes or most of the process outcomes measured in the study (Nielsen et al., 2007). Although the design of this study originally included both outcome analysis and assessment of the teamwork implementation process, the process assessment was dropped due to cutbacks in study funding. Therefore, the study could not assess how the participating hospitals implemented the teamwork practices in which they were trained. As a result, the authors did not have the information they needed in order to explore which factors might be related to the negative outcomes.

Nielsen et al. considered several possible explanations for these negative results, including ineffectiveness of the training, need for more-intensive training, inadequate time allowed for implementation of the practices learned, and inadequate timeline for observing outcome effects. Their subsequent experience in implementing teamwork indicated that nine to 12 months may be required before a significant decline in patient outcomes would be observable (Nielsen et al., 2007).

A central issue of the clinical trial study was that the intervention defined for the study was only the initial teamwork training (with no subsequent implementation support for the L&D units). This issue led to the following specific study design issues:

- After the teamwork training was completed, the intervention sites were left on their own to implement teamwork practices, with no training or support on the QI methods required to make improved teamwork a reality.
- The initial training also was not followed by any subsequent coaching or refresher training on the teamwork practices as the L&D units worked on implementing teamwork improvements.
- The absence of a process evaluation prevented the study team from observing and documenting the extent to which the intervention sites actually implemented teamwork practices following their training.
- Other possible outcomes were not examined, such as changes in care processes, efficiencies, or staff experiences.
- Trends in outcome measures tracked during the study were quite short, so they might not have captured changes in outcomes that require more time to become observable.

Overview of the Evaluation

The evaluation study presented in this report was designed to address the issues that may have contributed to the negative findings of the earlier study. The first three issues are related to the implementation work involved in achieving adoption of improved teamwork practices—lack of support as hospitals implemented teamwork practices, no coaching or refresher training, and absence of a process evaluation. The other two issues relate to limitations of the outcome analysis of effects of teamwork practices—outcome measures limited to patient outcomes and use of a short timeline for assessing changes in outcomes.

Quality-Improvement Framework

Our evaluation design was based on a QI framework. According to this framework, effective quality improvement comes about through regular, incremental changes in the practices of interest, guided by measurement, monitoring, and feedback on performance (Imai, 1986). Hundreds of articles have been published about specific QI applications for health-care services, which had varying levels of success in achieving their goals. Examples include applications in obstetric care, prescription drugs, primary-care services, emergency departments, radiology, and surgical care (Solberg et al., 1998; Cox, Wilcock, and Young, 1999; Glezerman et al., 1999; Schwab et al., 1999; Gandhi et al., 2000; Harris et al., 2000; Laurila et al., 2001). These experiences have shown consistently that effective implementation is the key to achieving performance improvements. A QI program needs to motivate the staff at each delivery site to plan, execute, and evaluate organizational change.

We combined the QI framework with a case-study approach that allowed us to embrace the natural variation in implementation activities across the participating L&D units, rather than attempting to have the L&D units implement the same intervention. The goal was for all the L&D units to fully implement all the practices included in the teamwork model. However, they were not "locked in" to a uniform set of steps for implementing the model and its specific teamwork practices. Each unit developed and carried out an implementation strategy that it felt worked best for its unit and team, one that would reflect its situation and performance issues.

In addition, we chose for participation in the study five L&D units that had made an explicit commitment to improving teamwork practices. We do not believe that this prevented us from examining the generalizability of the evaluation results to other L&D units. Rather, the reference group for generalizability consists of other units that also are committed to these changes. Our rationale is based on the general recognition in QI science that successful adoption of a new practice takes work and perseverance (Kuperman et al., 1991; Larson, 2002; Pronovost and Holzmueller, 2004), and those that do not persevere tend not to achieve improvements.

Relationship Between the Teamwork Implementation and Our Evaluation

We made a distinction between the implementation activities of the participating L&D units and the evaluation we conducted to learn from their experiences. The logic model in Figure 1.1 identifies the steps taken by the hospitals in implementing teamwork improvements and shows how our evaluation related to those activities. The middle row of the model (Hospital L&D units) represents a three-step sequence of teamwork status, starting with baseline status, moving to change in teamwork practices resulting from improvement activities, and ultimately leading to improved team-based care. The top row of the model represents the training provided, including the initial training of unit staff, follow-up coaching, and refresher training over time. Finally, the bottom row of the model represents the approach and data-collection schedule for our evaluation of the implementation process.

For our evaluation, we identified four research questions, two of which addressed each study objective (noted earlier at the beginning of this chapter and repeated below). The first

Figure 1.1
Evaluation Components for the Labor and Delivery Teamwork Implementation Study

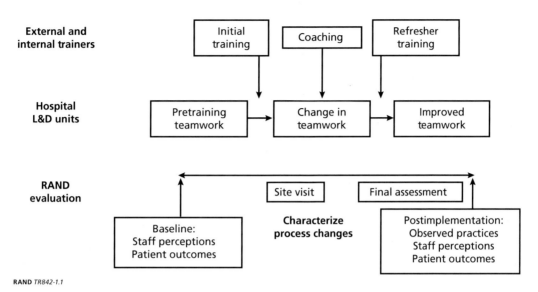

RAND *TR842-1.1*

objective was addressed by the process evaluation, and the second objective was addressed by the outcome evaluation.

- *Objective 1:* Better understand the conditions and actions required for hospital L&D units to achieve effective and sustainable teamwork practices, by asking the following research questions:
  - What training and actions are required to achieve a high level of teamwork in the L&D process?
  - How strongly do self-reported experiences in implementing teamwork improvements correlate with actual levels of teamwork as measured by direct observation of the L&D process?
- *Objective 2:* Assess the extent to which successful adoption of teamwork practices may influence the experiences of staff working in the units and outcomes for patients, by asking the following research questions:
  - How does achieving effective teamwork affect the perceptions and experiences of staff working in L&D units?
  - What effects does effective teamwork have on L&D outcomes for mothers and new-born infants?

A more detailed description of our study approach and methods appears in Chapter Two.

Organization of This Report

The remaining chapters of this report present the methods (Chapter Two), results (Chapters Three and Four), and conclusions (Chapter Five) of our evaluation. The process-evaluation results are presented in Chapter Three, and the outcome-evaluation results are presented in Chapter Four. The outcome-evaluation results include effects of teamwork implementation on staff working in the units, and effects on patient outcomes. Chapter Five presents a discussion of our results, draws conclusions from the study, and explores their implications.

CHAPTER TWO

Study Design and Methods

In this section, we describe in detail the design and methods used for evaluating teamwork practice implementation by the five participating L&D units. There were two parts to this evaluation: (1) a process evaluation of the implementation process itself and (2) an outcome evaluation of the effects that improved use of team-based care had on staff perceptions and knowledge and on patient outcomes.

We first present the conceptual model that guided our data collection and analysis for the evaluation, which is grounded in the principles of QI implementation processes. Then we give a brief overview of the evaluation design, derived from this model. Next, we describe how we selected the L&D units for the study and profile their characteristics. In the rest of the chapter, we present in detail the methods used for the process evaluation and outcome evaluation. Finally, we end the chapter with a discussion of the limitations of the evaluation.

Conceptual Model for Quality-Improvement Implementation

Hundreds of papers have been published that report results of health-care providers' QI efforts. Many of the same factors are reported repeatedly in these papers as having affected (either positively or negatively) the degree of success that organizations had in implementing the performance improvements they sought (for example, Alexander et al., 2006; Gross et al., 2001; Taylor et al., 2009).

Rycroft-Malone et al. (2002) developed a model that specifies that successful implementation of evidence-based care practice is a function of three core elements—the level and nature of the evidence for the practice, the context or environment into which implementation is to take place, and the methods used to facilitate the process. The models used by many QI experts (e.g., Institute for Healthcare Improvement) to guide QI activities are built on these elements.

The AHRQ TeamSTEPPS system also applies QI methods in its guidance to hospitals that are implementing TeamSTEPPS. On its TeamSTEPPS website, AHRQ states that a successful TeamSTEPPS initiative requires a thorough assessment of the organization and its processes and careful development of an implementation and sustainment plan (AHRQ, undated). To this end, it specifies the following phases for TeamSTEPPS adoption and provides guidance for carrying out each phase:

Phase 1. Assess the Need—determine an organization's readiness for undertaking a TeamSTEPPS-based initiative by performing a training needs analysis.

Phase 2. Planning, Training, and Implementation—carry out the training and implementation of teamwork tools and strategies, as determined most appropriate for the organization (from full implementation of all tools to partial implementation of some tools or in some departments; called a "dosing strategy" in TeamSTEPPS parlance), while maintaining the primary learning objectives.

Phase 3. Sustainment—sustain and spread improvements in teamwork performance, clinical processes, and outcomes resulting from the TeamSTEPPS initiative, by ensuring that opportunities exist to continue use of the tools and strategies taught, and provide continual reinforcement of the TeamSTEPPS principles, following the initial implementation activities. (AHRQ, undated)

The conceptual model we adopted for this evaluation encompasses the core elements involved in QI implementation, and it emphasizes stakeholders' role in the dynamics of the implementation process. This model was developed for use in evaluations of QI initiatives undertaken by providers to improve their performance on the Consumer Assessment of Healthcare Providers and Systems (CAHPS) survey, and it has been used in other studies (Farley et al., 2007). This framework, presented in Figure 2.1, consists of concentric levels of components, with stakeholders involved at two of those levels. At the center of the model is the intervention itself (in which the stakeholders are the implementation-team leads), team members, and other directly involved staff.

The intervention works within the organizational environment, including organizational philosophy and capacity. Stakeholders within this environment include executive leadership, as well as staff in other units or departments, whose responses to an intervention can affect its

Figure 2.1
Conceptual Model for a Quality-Improvement Initiative

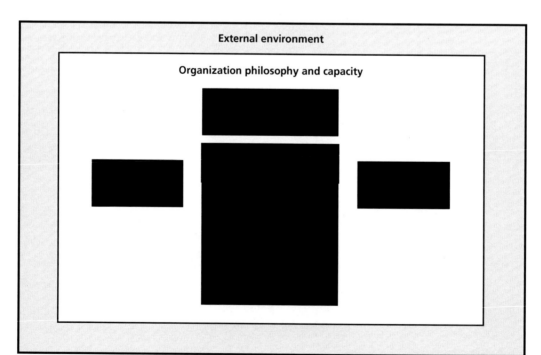

progress. In addition, patients and families are key stakeholders, as the people served by the organization, who likely vary in characteristics and preferences for care. Finally, the organization operates within a larger external environment, which may affect its activities either positively or negatively.

Information on each of the elements of this model was collected in the process evaluation by including questions on the interview protocols relevant to each element, including attention to the involvement and reactions of various stakeholder groups to the teamwork-practice implementation activities. We also examined which implementation actions were undertaken at different points of time during the implementation period. For example, we documented when and how the implementation team was organized, when training was provided and to whom, and when work was initiated on adopting the individual teamwork practices (see Table 1.1 in Chapter One).

Overview of the Evaluation Design

As described in Chapter One, each evaluation component was designed to collect and analyze data to address one of the two study objectives (see Table 2.1).

Both the process and outcome evaluations were essential to being able to achieve our study goals of understanding the dynamics of the teamwork-improvement process and how that process ultimately affects desired outcomes. By tracking the activities of the L&D units throughout a one-year study period and examining effects of those activities on staff and patient outcomes, we could assess which structures and processes may be needed to achieve teamwork improvements and outcome effects. The data-collection components and schedule are summarized in Table 2.2. Details of the methods used are described later in this chapter.

We started data collection on different dates for each participating hospital, depending on when the L&D unit scheduled its initial staff training on teamwork skills and practices and when it obtained approval from its hospital institutional review board (IRB) to participate in the study. Thus, each L&D unit had its own implementation year. We started to collect process evaluation and staff survey data for all of the L&D units except one in the spring and summer of 2006—two in March 2006, one in April 2006, and one in July 2006. The last L&D units experienced a delay in obtaining hospital IRB approval, as a result of which we started data collection in July 2007; however, they already had collected baseline staff survey data for their own use, which they provided to us as soon as they obtained the IRB approval. To perform our analyses, we anchored the start dates for all the L&D units as month 1 of implementation and defined timelines relative to that month.

Table 2.1
Evaluation Components Addressing Study Objectives

Study Objective	Evaluation Component
Better understand the conditions and actions required for hospital L&D units to achieve effective and sustainable teamwork practices.	Process evaluation
Assess the extent to which successful adoption of teamwork practices may influence the experiences of staff working in the units and outcomes for patients.	Outcome evaluation

Table 2.2
Schedule of Evaluation Data-Collection Activities

| | Timing Relative to Implementation Year | | |
Activity	Baseline	Early	Late
Process evaluation			
Group interviews		Site visit	Final assessment
Update calls		Monthly	
Direct observation			x
Outcome evaluation			
staff survey	x		x
Patient outcomes[a]	x	x	x

[a] Patient outcomes were measured on a quarterly basis.

The process evaluation documented the extent to which the L&D units implemented teamwork training, took advantage of coaching, began other initiatives, or experienced disruptions that might affect process and outcome measures. A site visit to each L&D unit was conducted early in its implementation activities, which allowed us to document and gain insights into each unit's early implementation experiences. At the close of the data-collection period, we conducted a final assessment via a two-hour teleconference, in which we gathered data from the implementation teams on the status of each L&D unit and lessons learned after a year of activity. Throughout the study year, we conducted monthly telephone update interviews with the leads of the units' implementation teams to obtain close-to-real-time data on their progress at different points in time. We used the process-evaluation data to document the evolution of their teamwork-improvement activities, successes achieved, challenges encountered, and the pace at which they adopted the specific teamwork practices delineated in either the MedTeams or TeamSTEPPS curriculum. Finally, their self-reported teamwork status at the end of the study was compared with data collected in an observation study, also conducted at the end of the study.

In the outcome evaluation, we analyzed two categories of outcomes—patient-safety knowledge and perceptions of the staff working in the L&D units, and adverse outcomes experienced by mothers and infants served by the units. Data for measuring staff perceptions and knowledge, and changes in them over time, were collected in a staff survey conducted twice during the study period. To estimate effects on patients, we used the L&D outcome measures developed as part of the previous L&D study funded by DoD (Mann et al., 2006), which include sets of measures for maternal outcomes and newborn outcomes. The National Perinatal Information Center (NPIC) calculated hospital-level rates for these measures on a quarterly basis, using hospital discharge data provided to it by the participating hospitals.

Selection of the Participating Labor and Delivery Units

The hospitals that participated in this study were a subset of the 15 hospitals that were involved in the original Labor and Delivery Teamwork Intervention Trial conducted by Nielsen and associates (2007). To identify candidates for participation, we conducted a brief interview with the study lead for each hospital, in which we asked about efforts they had undertaken since the previous study to implement teamwork improvements and inquired about their interest in participating in this follow-up study.

Our goal was to identify five L&D units from the original study in which the leadership of the units had made a commitment to strengthen their teamwork practices and either had begun or planned to move forward with QI interventions to do so. In particular, we wanted the sample to consist of three civilian and two military hospitals so we could compare experiences across these two sectors. We also sought to include both teaching and nonteaching hospitals. Ideally, all of the hospitals would have been in the control group of the original study, so that we would be able to observe early experiences from their improvement processes.

The hospital L&D units that participated in the study are listed in Table 2.3. All of the L&D units included in the study expressed their commitment to strengthening their teamwork practices, and they stated that they would have pursued this goal even in the absence of our evaluation. We achieved the civilian-military mix we sought, as well as the desired variation in teaching status for the civilian hospitals.

We were not able to limit the participants to those in the original control group, however, for a variety of reasons, including limited implementation activity and lack of interest in the study. As a result, the participating hospitals were at varying stages of progress in implementing teamwork improvements at the start of the study. Some already had made progress in enhancing teamwork skills and practices, while others were just beginning their work. Although this created some challenges for making accurate comparisons across L&D units, it provided a breadth of experience across a longer implementation timeline that enriched the lessons we could draw from the study.

We took these differences into account in both the collection and analysis of the data, as discussed later for each component of the evaluation methodology. For the process evaluation, differences in practice-implementation status reflected both the extent of work performed before our study started and the pace (intensity) of implementation during the study. We adjusted for these differences by developing a timeline for each L&D unit that documented when it implemented each teamwork practice and anchoring the timeline on the month it started the implementation process (as month 1). For the outcome evaluations, we established a threshold month that separated the baseline and implementation periods for purposes of

Table 2.3
Hospital Labor and Delivery Units Participating in This Study

Labor and Delivery Unit	Status in Original Study	Type of Hospital	Deliveries in 2004
Site 1	Control	Civilian, community	4,000
Site 2	Control	Civilian, academic	1,705
Site 3	Intervention	Civilian, teaching	6,700
Site 4	Intervention	Military	3,600
Site 5	Control	Military	3,000

NOTE: An academic hospital is one that is an integral part of a university and medical-school teaching program. A teaching hospital is a community hospital with a residency program. A community hospital does not have any medical training program.

our modeling analysis. This threshold for each L&D unit was placed at the time that the unit started the teamwork training for its staff at the start of this study. Our interpretation of the outcome trends for each unit took into account both this threshold and the existence of team-work-implementation activities that predated that threshold.

Human-Subject Protection Requirements

All the components of the evaluation study were reviewed and approved by the RAND Human Subjects Protection Committee (RAND's IRB), including annual update reviews to ensure compliance with informed consent and data privacy requirements. The study also was reviewed and approved by the IRBs for DoD's TRICARE Management Activity (TMA) and each of the five participating hospitals. The TMA IRB reviewed the project because TMA funded the work, and the hospital IRBs reviewed it because they were participants in the study. The hospital IRBs required reviews even though the hospital L&D units were performing the QI activities and were the subjects of the RAND study (i.e., not performing the research), which reflected the careful approach that many health-care organizations are taking for human-subject protection and informed consent in health-care research.

Process-Evaluation Methods

As described earlier, the process evaluation was designed to address the first objective of the study and the associated two research questions. The process evaluation addressed each research question, as indicated in Table 2.4.

Longitudinal Assessment of Teamwork-Implementation Activities

We developed the data-collection methods for the teamwork-implementation activities to capture data on each of the activities typically involved in implementing teamwork-improvement strategies and interventions (which also apply more generally to most QI activities). The L&D unit began by identifying the need for improvement and making a commitment to pursuing actions to address it, which the participating units had done before the study started. Then the units established implementation or leadership teams, which developed and carried out a strategy for actions to improve teamwork practices. The goal of the implementation activities

Table 2.4
Process Evaluation: Better Understand the Conditions and Actions Required for Hospital Labor and Delivery Units to Achieve Effective and Sustainable Teamwork Practices

Research Question	Method
What training and actions are required to achieve a high level of teamwork in the L&D process?	Collect and analyze longitudinal qualitative data on the implementation activities carried out by the participating L&D units to assess their progress and experiences in achieving teamwork improvements.
How strongly do self-reported experiences in implementing teamwork improvements correlate with actual levels of teamwork as measured by direct observation of the L&D process?	Directly observe teamwork practices in the L&D units at the end of the observed implementation period to assess their status at that time and relate it to data on their implementation activities and on staff perceptions.

undertaken by the L&D units was to institutionalize the improved teamwork practices so that strong, team-based care became an integral part of how the L&D units "do business."

The first step in the process of implementing teamwork-practice improvements in each L&D unit was to provide training on teamwork practices and skills for L&D staff, including physicians, nurses, other clinical staff, and clerical staff. All five units conducted teamwork training for the staff at the start of this study, including those who already had received training as part of the earlier clinical-trial study. The training was followed by active interventions by the units' implementation teams to encourage staff to use these practices and skills as they serve patients in the unit. These interventions included ongoing coaching and reinforcement, including refresher training as needed.

We chose a mix of methods to collect data that would give us as clear a perspective as possible on how the L&D units undertook each of these activities and their experiences in carrying out the work. We used this rich information to examine the research question of what training and actions are required to achieve a high level of teamwork in L&D. We also used it to help interpret findings from the outcome evaluation about effects that the implementation activities had on staff and patients. We describe here each of the data-collection methods used.

Site Visits to the L&D Units. Within three to four months after each L&D unit performed its initial teamwork training, we conducted an on-site evaluation visit to the unit. Each site visit lasted one day, during which we conducted a series of individual and group interviews with the leaders of the teamwork initiative, the implementation team, and other affected stakeholder groups. The site visits served the following purposes:

- to gain an understanding of the unit's dynamics and care processes, which served as context to help us interpret the data collected during the process evaluation
- to gather qualitative data on the unit's experiences during its planning and early implementation of teamwork-improvement strategies
- to document and compare the perspectives and experiences of the various groups of stakeholders, and variations across them, regarding the teamwork-improvement activities.

For each L&D unit, we worked with the implementation lead to develop the itinerary for the site visit, and the lead then recruited participants for each of the scheduled interviews. Group interviews were conducted with the implementation team, as well as three other stakeholder groups—physicians, nurses, and other clinic staff. We also did individual interviews with the lead staff and higher-level management personnel when we were able to schedule them.

All the interviews were guided by written protocols with questions and probes for topics we wanted to address with each individual or group. We developed a matrix consisting of a master list of topics and related questions, along with notations that identified the stakeholder groups that should be asked each question (see Appendix B). The questions in the matrix related to the following major topic areas:

- hospital environment for quality and safety
- patient-safety culture in the L&D unit
- hospital leadership support for L&D teamwork
- the teamwork-improvement team
- teamwork training for the L&D unit staff

- implementing teamwork improvements
- assessment of L&D teamwork performance
- concluding summary questions on insights gained from experience.

From this matrix, we then created separate interview protocols that contained the relevant questions for each of four groups—implementation team and leads, physicians and midwives, nurses, and clerical staff.

We were able to complete the site visits for three civilian hospitals early in their implementation period, as planned, but we could not do so for the two military hospitals due to delays in obtaining approvals from their hospital IRBs. We conducted the visits at the military hospitals approximately ten months after they performed their initial training. To adjust for the delay in these site visits, we included questions in the interviews with them that probed the history of their implementation activities and related effects on stakeholders. Although data from visits to the military hospitals are vulnerable to recall bias because respondents were reporting on past activities, we obtained useful information from them on the evolution of their implementation experiences. We took this issue into account in our interpretation of the process-evaluation results.

Monthly Update Telephone Meetings with Team Leads. The purpose of the monthly update telephone meetings was to capture in near-real time the evolution of the teamwork implementation activities and related experiences, which could not have been captured as accurately in post hoc interviews due to incomplete or inaccurate participant recall. These teleconferences were held with the key leads for each L&D unit. We developed a monthly update teleconference worksheet (see Appendix C) that listed the topics to be addressed in each monthly discussion. This worksheet was provided to the unit leads with whom we talked, so that we all worked from the same reference material. The emphasis of discussion varied over time, depending on the current status of each unit in its implementation process, and we decided together with them which topics should be the focus of each discussion. These monthly discussions yielded important factual data on the timeline of specific activities for the implementation process, as well as on the successes and challenges experienced as the teamwork-improvement efforts moved forward. For example, each unit lead identified several successes and challenges each month, but the nature of those successes and challenges changed over time.

Final-Assessment Telephone Interviews. At the end of the study year, we closed the evaluation by conducting a two-hour telephone interview with each L&D unit, in which we asked the participants to share their views and lessons learned as they looked back over their experiences in implementing improved teamwork practices. Some of the L&D units used this interview as an opportunity to engage their full implementation teams in the review of their experiences and progress. Again, we developed a written protocol to guide the discussion, which we shared with the unit leads in advance, to help them prepare for the interview (see Appendix D). At the start of the interview, we asked them to envision that they were advising other L&D unit teams that were about to embark upon the same journey that they had just pursued.

Analysis of Implementation Assessment Results. The qualitative data collected during the site visits and teleconferences with the sites consisted of both factual information on the steps taken for implementation of the teamwork practices and experiential information on the dynamics of the implementation process and how it affected various stakeholders. Using standard case-study analysis methods (Miles and Huberman, 1994; Strauss and Corbin, 1998;

Ryan and Bernard, 2000), we developed a timeline for each site that showed when it carried out each key implementation action. These actions included the organization and operation of their implementation teams, provision of initial and follow-up training to unit staff, the introduction of each teamwork practice, and the ultimate integration of each practice into the unit's care processes. We also identified common themes and variations in experiences that could help guide similar work by other L&D units, by summarizing the experiential information provided by the sites for each question on the interview protocol.

We considered the factual and experiential process-evaluation results together to assess the overall progress of each site in achieving its teamwork-improvement goals and to identify factors contributing to that progress. We reviewed our data on the experiences of the five sites to identify common themes, as well as differences in patterns of actions and dynamics across sites. The focus of this portion of the analysis was on the successes and challenges reported by the sites, together with feedback from stakeholder groups interviewed during the site visits. The challenges were classified as either actions or events resulting from teamwork implementation (internal challenges) or actions or events that originated from outside the unit that affected their progress (external challenges).

Direct Observations of Teamwork Practices in Care Delivery

One round of direct observations was conducted in each L&D unit at the end of the study, immediately preceding our conduct of the final-assessment telephone interview for the unit. The purpose of the observation studies was to obtain direct information regarding the level of teamwork practices in each unit across four TeamSTEPPS competencies—leadership, situation monitoring, mutual support, and communication—plus a fifth dimension of team structure.

The teamwork practices of each L&D unit were rated using the Team Performance Observation Tool and the accompanying behaviorally anchored rating scale (BARS) (see Appendix E).

- The *observation tool* provides a worksheet format on which ratings of observed performance are recorded on a five-point scale for each of the teamwork competency areas and subtopics within them.
- The *BARS* delineates the sets of behaviors that comprise effective teamwork on each of these five competency areas and provides guidance regarding which behaviors are associated with superior, acceptable, or very poor ratings.

The focus of the direct observations was the staff activities at and around the central nursing station in the L&D unit. The interactions of the delivery staff during these clinical processes were documented and rated based on how effectively staff used teamwork practices. No observations were conducted of any interactions between the staff and individual patients, and no information about individual patients was recorded in the observation notes.

The observations were performed by one observer who is clinically trained as a registered nurse (RN), is an expert and trainer on health-care teamwork practices, and has extensive experience in observation methods and practice. This individual performed a total of 12 hours of observations during three four-hour observation periods at each L&D unit. The first period was four hours during an evening shift, the second was four hours that included a hand-off from evening to night shift, and the third period was four hours that include a hand-off from night to day shifts.

The unit of observation for the teamwork-practice assessments was a one-hour time period. For each hour of observation, the observer rated a unit's performance on each aspect of teamwork listed in the observation form, using a five-point scale (where 1 = very poor and 5 = excellent). Over the total observation time in an L&D unit, 12 one-hour rating data points were generated for each of 25 elements, grouped in the five dimensions of teamwork practices (see Appendix E). The observer also prepared qualitative notes regarding specific actions, practices, and issues observed during each period. Both the ratings and observation notes were reported back to the L&D unit's leadership to provide feedback to help the unit strengthen its practices. Because this feedback was provided at the end of the study, it did not affect the implementation progress being documented during the process evaluation.

Analysis of the Observation Data. Using the rating data, we calculated average ratings and assessed the extent of variation in teamwork performance for the teamwork dimensions, both within each L&D unit and across units. Because only one person performed all the observation studies at all the participating L&D units, we were able to achieve consistent (reliable) observation ratings.

The observer and the evaluation team examined the observation results, including average ratings and variations in ratings across sites and teamwork dimensions, and compared these results to the self-reported information on the units' practice implementation from the process evaluation. Where the observation results for an L&D unit appeared to differ from what was learned in the process evaluation, the observation results helped to inform our interpretation of the process-evaluation results. None of the observation scores was changed as a result of this analysis.

Outcome-Evaluation Methods

As described earlier, the outcome evaluation was designed to address the second objective of the study and the associated two research questions. The outcome evaluation addressed each research question as outlined in Table 2.5.

In the outcome evaluation, we examined effects of the teamwork improvements pursued by the L&D units on both proximal and distal outcomes. The proximal outcomes were effects on staff perceptions and knowledge regarding teamwork culture and practices, with the expectation that, as staff gain new knowledge and skills, these changes should be measurable in staff survey data. The more-distal effects were effects on patient outcomes for mothers and infants. Because the patient outcomes tend to be adverse events of low frequency, these effects required observation over longer timeframes to detect events. Therefore, more data over time

Table 2.5
Outcome Evaluation: Assess the Extent to Which Successful Adoption of Teamwork Practices May Influence the Experiences of Staff Working in the Units and Outcomes for Patients

Research Question	Method
How does achieving effective teamwork affect the patient-safety perceptions, experiences, and knowledge of staff working in L&D units?	Analyze survey data on staff perceptions of teamwork in the units, collected at two points in time during the implementation period we observed (early and late).
What effects does effective teamwork have on L&D outcomes for mothers and newborn infants?	Analyze trends in outcomes for patients of the L&D units in order to assess relationships between these outcomes and the implementation activities and staff perceptions.

are required to estimate meaningful event rates and to identify statistically significant changes in those rates.

Effects on Staff Perceptions and Knowledge of Teamwork

We examined three aspects of L&D staff perceptions about teamwork, which might change in response to teamwork-practice improvement:

- staff knowledge of teamwork practices and skills
- staff perceptions of teamwork in the units
- work experiences of staff in the units.

The data for these analyses were collected in a survey of the staff working in the L&D units. Questions included in the survey addressed several aspects of teamwork, which are shown in Table 2.6. The questionnaire is provided in Appendix F. The survey items are organized into five major topic areas: hospital-level culture of patient safety, unit-level culture of patient safety, teamwork in L&D, quality of work life, and knowledge of teamwork. The survey took approximately 8 minutes to complete.

Table 2.6
Dimensions Covered in the Staff Survey Questionnaire

Survey Dimension	Number of Items[a]	Source Survey
Hospital-level culture of patient safety		
Hospital management support for patient safety	3	HSOPS
Hospital hand-offs and transitions	2 of 4	HSOPS
Organizational learning: continuous improvement	3	HSOPS
Teamwork across hospital units	1 of 4	HSOPS
Culture of patient safety in L&D		
Patient-safety grade	1	HSOPS
Nonpunitive response to error	3	HSOPS
Overall patient-safety status in the unit	4	HSOPS
Patient-safety climate in the unit	5 of 7	SAQ
Teamwork in L&D		
Teamwork within the unit	4	HSOPS
Communication openness	3	HSOPS
Teamwork climate	2 of 6	SAQ
Quality of work life[b]	6	Self-developed
Knowledge of teamwork	8	Self-developed

NOTE: HSOPS = Hospital Survey on Patient Safety Culture. SAQ = Safety Attitude Questionnaire.
[a] For some dimensions, a subset of the items in either the HSOPS or SAQ was used for this survey.
[b] Two of the six items in this dimension are taken from the SAQ.

The Survey Questionnaire. With the exception of two content dimensions, the survey items were drawn from existing, well-tested survey instruments, so their psychometric properties were known. The source surveys were HSOPS and the SAQ (Sorra and Nieva, 2004; Sexton et al., 2004). As shown in Table 2.6, we used all of the questions from the source surveys for seven of the dimensions and subsets of questions for the other four dimensions. The questions dropped were those deemed to be the least relevant to the content of the teamwork-improvement work being undertaken by the L&D units in the study. This approach allowed us to keep the survey as short as possible, to encourage response rates, while retaining the most-relevant questions.

The six items in the quality-of-work-life dimension include two items from the SAQ survey plus four items written by our evaluation team that we felt addressed work life for staff in L&D units more closely than did other items available in the SAQ. We estimated correlation coefficients between each of these individual items and the composite measure calculated for the quality-of-work-life dimension and the composite measures for the other dimensions the survey covered. The results presented in Table 2.7 show that all of the individual items correlated most strongly with the quality-of-work-life dimension (shown in bold), with weaker correlations with composites for the other dimensions, indicating that they perform well as a composite.

The knowledge-of-teamwork items were used to measure the L&D staff's level of knowledge of teamwork principles and practices. Working in collaboration with the staff of the TMA Office of Patient Safety, we wrote eight multiple-choice questions that addressed various aspects of the teamwork practices that were taught in the MedTeams or TeamSTEPPS training. For analysis of results, an individual's response to each of these questions was coded as a dichotomous variable (1 = correct, 0 = incorrect).

Survey Data Collection. The staff survey was administered twice at each L&D unit during the study. For each survey administration, all staff currently working in an L&D unit were asked to complete the survey. Therefore, the baseline and follow-up survey samples for each unit were separate cross-sectional samples, i.e., we did not track one cohort of staff from baseline to the follow-up survey.

Results were used to analyze baseline staff perceptions and knowledge, as well as changes in perceptions or knowledge that took place during the period in which the participating L&D units were implementing their teamwork improvements. The baseline data for the study were collected immediately before the L&D units provided the initial teamwork training to their staff. We note that this was not the absolute baseline for those units that already had done some work on implementing teamwork practices. However, it was the baseline for this study because our goal was to assess how implementation activities that the units undertook during the study year may have affected their staff. The second data collection was performed at the end of the study year, which captured perceptions and knowledge after a year of improvement activities.

We originally planned to field online surveys that respondents could complete by logging into a web-based instrument. This approach failed to yield sufficient responses, so we switched to paper mode and distribution of the surveys to staff at organized meetings. The only exception was at one L&D unit that used its own internal web-based survey system to collect data for its follow-up survey, which yielded close to a 25-percent response rate. For all the other units, the data were collected using paper surveys. Completion of the surveys was voluntary, as explained in the consent language provided at the beginning of the questionnaire. We collaborated with our field partners in the L&D units in the data-collection process. The RAND

Table 2.7
Correlations of the Items in the Quality-of-Work-Life Composite to Each Composite in the Labor and Delivery Unit Staff Survey

Culture and Teamwork Domains	Item in Job-Satisfaction Domain					
	This Hospital Is a Good Place to Work	Morale in This Unit Is High	Operating Problems in the Unit Keep Me from Performing My Best	I Feel Like a Respected Member of the Team in the Unit	I Would Rather Not Be Working on This Unit	My Job Is Fulfilling Professionally
Work-life quality	0.695	0.635	0.592	0.680	0.627	0.591
Hospital management support for patient safety	0.327	0.247	0.186	0.205	0.158	0.172
Organizational learning: continuous improvement	0.331	0.285	0.201	0.236	0.225	0.212
Patient-safety grade	0.270	0.319	0.268	0.188	0.195	0.174
Nonpunitive response to error	0.111	0.174	0.222	0.186	0.146	0.050
Overall patient-safety status in unit	0.265	0.306	0.389	0.220	0.248	0.086
Teamwork within the unit	0.311	0.335	0.207	0.429	0.310	0.210
Communication openness	0.097	0.211	0.096	0.168	0.096	0.095

NOTE: Correlations were calculated only for domains that were composites of more than one item.

team provided the contact person at each hospital with the paper questionnaires, which he or she distributed to the staff in the L&D unit. The contact persons shipped the completed surveys to RAND, and we entered the data into electronic files for analysis.

The response rates varied across the participating L&D units, as reported in Table 2.8. Response rates tended to be higher for the baseline survey than the end-of-study survey.

Analysis of Survey Results. Guided by the study objective and associated research question, we examined baseline levels and changes in staff knowledge of teamwork practices and in staff perceptions regarding the effectiveness of teamwork in their units. Through the questions on quality of work life, we also examined how teamwork effectiveness was affecting their job experiences. The results of these analyses are presented in Chapter Four.

Because the baseline and follow-up survey data were for separate cross-sectional samples of staff, we could not calculate changes in scores for individual survey respondents. Therefore, our analyses of change in the teamwork and culture dimensions were at the aggregate level of averages for each L&D unit (not individual staff level). This also affected our specification and analyses of the regression equations for staff survey analyses, which are described next.

We developed a total of 13 measures that we grouped within the five major aspects of staff perceptions—hospital-level culture of patient safety, patient-safety culture in the L&D unit, teamwork in the L&D unit, quality of work life, and knowledge of teamwork. Two of these measures (teamwork across hospital units and patient-safety grade) were single items; the remaining 11 measures were composites based on more than one survey item.

To calculate each composite, we first assigned survey questions to each of the dimensions of interest (based on assignments made in the source surveys), and we identified questions with reverse wording. For each respondent, we counted the number of questions in each dimension for which the respondent had a positive response. Using the method recommended for HSOPS, we defined a positive response as a response in either of the top two response categories. For each respondent, we calculate a composite for each dimension, which is the number of positive responses to questions included in the dimension divided by the total number of questions in the dimension that the respondent answered. This generates the proportion of positive responses to questions in the domain that the respondent answered. Thus, questions that the respondent did not answer are excluded from the calculation of the composite.

Table 2.8
Response Rates for the Participating Labor and Delivery Units, Staff Surveys at Baseline and End of Study

L&D Unit	Number of Staff (denominator)	Baseline		End of Study	
		Completed Surveys	Response Rate (%)	Completed Surveys	Response Rate (%)
Site 1	225/208[a]	221	98.2	49	23.6
Site 2	142	72	50.7	75	52.8
Site 3	265	86	32.5	55	20.8
Site 4	108	32	29.6	43	39.8
Site 5	120	43	35.8	19	15.8

[a] The number of staff in this unit decreased from 225 to 208 during the study period. Staffing for the other four units remained fairly constant, so the same denominator was used to calculate response rates for both surveys.

High rates of missing values can affect the validity of values calculated for multi-item domains. Missing data was not a problem for this analysis, however, because rates of missing data for individual items were quite low. Missing-data rates for individual items ranged from 0.1 percent to 5.3 percent, and 73 percent of the items in the staff perception domains had less than 4.0 percent of the data missing. The items on teamwork knowledge with missing data were scored as incorrect answers, assuming that staff would have answered the question if they had known the answers.

As a first analytic step, we used the staff survey results for these 13 measures to develop an aggregate baseline profile of the staff perceptions, knowledge, and work life, and changes in those values, across all the participating L&D units. We then examined variations across units in the five domains covered in the survey, and changes in them over time, to compare these results with what we learned from the process evaluation about the baseline teamwork status and implementation activities of the units.

In these analyses, we tested our basic hypotheses that teamwork improvements in the L&D units should have the greatest effects on staff perceptions about teamwork on the unit, the quality of their work lives, and staff knowledge of teamwork practices. Improvements might also affect staff perceptions of patient-safety culture on the unit and, to a lesser extent, perceptions of patient-safety culture at the hospital level.

We also performed a series of regression analyses to estimate the factors contributing to changes in staff perceptions regarding teamwork in the L&D unit. Three measures fall within this domain—teamwork on the L&D unit, communication openness on the unit, and teamwork climate on the unit. Separate regressions were estimated for each of these measures as the dependent variables for the models. The independent variables in the regressions included dummy variables for sites; dummy variables for whether a site had implemented three or more teamwork practices, whether the site had done active coaching, and whether the site had a facilitator and trained all staff (implementation variables); survey wave (first or second); and respondent characteristics (time on unit, clinical status, and full-time or other). Changes in dependent variable were captured in the survey-wave variable.

Four different regression models were estimated for each of the three dependent variables. The first regression included independent variables for just the survey wave and site, the second added respondent characteristics, and the third added interaction terms for survey wave and site to detect differences across sites in survey responses over time. In the fourth model, we added the three implementation variables and removed the interaction terms for survey wave and site. This final model allowed us to examine the effects of implementation actions on staff perceptions.

All regressions clustered observations on site, adjusting standard errors to account for the lack of independence that would occur if the same individual participated in both waves of the survey (which, due to the anonymous nature of the survey, we could not assess), and used robust standard errors, which accommodates the presence of heteroskedasticity. We also tested for multicollinearity by assessing the variance inflation factor for each independent variable and evidence of omitted variables using the Ramsey test (Stata Corporation, 2003).

Effects on Patient Outcomes

Our analysis of the effects of teamwork improvements on patient outcomes used the ten patient-outcome measures developed in the original L&D teamwork trial, as well as the Adverse Outcome Indexes (AOIs) developed based on these measures (Mann et al., 2006). Using an expert consensus method, that study selected individual maternal and newborn outcome measures from a larger set of candidate measures. In making the selections, the participating experts considered several criteria for measure validity and relevance, as well as data on the frequency of occurrence of events that a measure addressed. The criteria applied to each candidate measure were (1) extent of support in the literature that the measure was a measure of quality, (2) ability to universally apply the measure to different practice environments, (3) precision of the definition of the measure, (4) significance of the frequency or severity of events the measure addressed, (5) reasonable feasibility for estimating the measure empirically, and (6) potential for improved teamwork to affect the measure. A workbook with precise definitions for each selected measure was created (Mann et al., 2006). The ten measures established are listed in Table 2.9.

Recognizing that the prevalence of each individual outcome measure is likely to be very low, the expert panel combined the outcome measures into an AOI. The AOI is a rate that is defined as the number of deliveries that had one or more of the identified outcomes divided by the total number of deliveries.

While the AOI gives a measure of frequency of deliveries with adverse events, it does not capture the severity of these outcomes. To assess the overall significance of events on an L&D unit, a Weighted Adverse Outcome Score (WAOS) was developed that weighted each outcome measure by a weight that represented the severity of the outcome (see Table 2.9). The American College of Obstetricians and Gynecologists' Committee on Patient Safety and Quality Improvement developed the weights using a consensus process. It was decided at the start of the process that the sum of the scores of all other outcomes could not be greater than the score

Table 2.9
Measures of Maternal and Neonate Outcomes Used to Assess Effects of Teamwork on Patient Outcomes

L&D Patient-Outcome Measure	Weight Applied to Adverse Outcome to Calculate WAOS
Maternal outcome measures	
Maternal deaths	750
Uterine rupture	100
Unplanned maternal admission to ICU	65
Return to OR/L&D	40
3rd- or 4th-degree perineal laceration	5
Maternal blood transfusion	20
Neonate outcome measures	
Intrapartum neonatal death >2,500 grams	400
Birth trauma	60
Admission to NICU of inborn neonate of >2,500 grams and ≥37 weeks gestation	35
Apgar <7 at 5 minutes for neonate ≥2,500 grams	25

SOURCE: Mann et al. (2006).

NOTE: ICU = intensive-care unit. OR = operating room. NICU = neonatal intensive-care unit. Apgar is an index used to evaluate a newborn's condition.

for a maternal death (Mann et al., 2006). The WAOS is defined as the sum of the adverse outcome scores of all events divided by the total number of deliveries. In addition, a severity index (SI) is calculated by dividing the same sum of scores by the number of patients with one or more adverse events. The SI measures the average severity of the adverse events experienced.

Obtaining and Use of the Adverse Outcome Index Data

To develop data on these outcome measures for this study, the participating L&D units provided their hospital-discharge data to NPIC, which estimated rates for each individual measure and the AOI, WAOS, and SI. NPIC provided the results to the participating L&D units for use in monitoring effects of their teamwork-improvement interventions, as well as to RAND for our outcome analysis.

NPIC calculated the hospital-level rates for these measures on a quarterly basis. Our goal was to establish outcome trends that were as long as possible, to give us the best chance of observing changes in patient outcomes for the hospitals and to relate these outcomes to the L&D units' teamwork-improvement activities. We took this approach to address one of the limitations of the original study: that the time from the start of implementation to the end of the study was too short to capture possible longer-term effects on outcomes. The timelines for the patient-outcome trends analyzed are presented in Table 2.10. The time-specific threshold points we established for each hospital to separate baseline from implementation time periods (shown in Table 2.10 as S) were anchored by their calendar of initial training dates.

The different timelines for the participating hospitals, shown in Table 2.10, reflect the times at which they carried out their teamwork-implementation activities. For example, two hospitals were somewhat slow to engage in the training and teamwork implementation because of staffing constraints. Another hospital proceeded at a gradual pace. We obtained data for these three hospitals all the way through calendar year 2007 to allow more time for effects to be observed.

Analysis of the Adverse Outcome Index Trend Data

We performed a descriptive analysis of the effects of teamwork improvement on patient outcomes by observing the trends in both the AOIs and WAOSs for each of the participating

Table 2.10
Timelines of Data Used for Estimating Trends in Patient-Outcome Measures

Participating L&D Unit	2005				2006				2007			
	Q1	Q2	Q3	Q4	Q1	Q2	Q3	Q4	Q1	Q2	Q3	Q4
Site 1	x	x	x	x	x	S	x	x	x	x		
Site 2	x	x	x	x	S	x	x	x	x	x	x	
Site 3	x	x	x	x	x	S	x	x	x	x	x	x
Site 4	x	x	x	x	x	x	S	x	x	x	x	x
Site 5	x	x	x	x	x	x	S	x	x	x	x	x

NOTE: An S signifies the quarter in which the L&D unit conducted its initial staff training and started teamwork-improvement implementation. Quarters preceding this time represent the baseline period used for each L&D unit to analyze effects of teamwork improvement on patient outcomes.

L&D units. We graphed those trends to identify any observed changes in trends between the baseline and implementation periods. Results of these analyses are reported in Chapter Four.

We also estimated a grouped logistic regression for each site separately to assess the relationship between the unit's AOI scores and the teamwork training and implementation that it performed. All analyses were performed using Stata version 9.0. We used a piecewise linear function for time with a single knot (i.e., two linear segments) denoting the quarter in which the teamwork training took place (Gould, 1993; Greene, 2003; Panis, 1994). We used two formulations, which allowed us to assess whether AOI scores changed, as well as the effect that the training itself might have had on any identified changes:

1. The quarter in which teamwork training was implemented was included in the second segment (i.e., the teamwork training quarter was included in the post period, under the assumption that its effect would be immediate).
2. The quarter in which teamwork training was implemented was included in the first segment (i.e., the teamwork training quarter was included in the pre period, under the assumption that its effect would not be immediate).

Limitations of the Evaluation

The multifaceted design of the evaluation is one of its key strengths because it provides several different data sources that can be used to generate a robust assessment of teamwork-implementation experiences and effects both on staff working in the units and on the patients they serve. Thus, this study addressed one of the shortcomings of the original L&D teamwork study—lack of information on the teamwork-implementation process that could be used to interpret findings on patient outcomes. However, this study also had some limitations that affected the extent to which we could interpret effects on the outcomes we examined, several of which were due to budget constraints.

Case studies yielded rich information on the dynamics of implementation processes, but there is some uncertainty regarding the extent to which these results can be generalized to a larger population of L&D units. If sufficient consistency is found in the themes that emerged from the process evaluation, the important factors identified can be interpreted with some confidence as likely being relevant for others as well. However, it is possible that, if other L&D units were observed as additional case studies, some different factors or strategies might emerge that also influence implementation success.

The group to which these results will be relevant is other L&D units that are motivated enough to persevere in implementing changes to culture and practices that are required to achieve sustainable team-based care. Given the difficulty involved in implementing effective team-based care, those that are not motivated are not likely to make much progress toward that end. It was for this reason that, for our study, we selected L&D units that were so motivated.

We considered the sites' implementation experiences to be "best-case" situations because of their commitment to improvement and their involvement in our study. They were involved in our data-collection processes, including the monthly update calls, site visits, observation studies, staff surveys, and final-assessment interviews. The questions we asked prompted them to think about issues they otherwise might not have considered. We received feedback from several unit leaders that our study activities helped to keep them focused on the teamwork-improvement work. This dynamic is a Hawthorne effect, but it also may be viewed as a proxy for the structure and discipline that L&D units need to impose on themselves to establish an accountability mechanism that keeps them on track.

In the original study design, we had planned to do a two-year longitudinal design. This was not possible, however, because we could not obtain the funding to support the second year of the research. This limited our ability to detect later implementation actions that were important to ultimate adoption success, or to detect effects on the outcomes that might require more than one year to become observable.

Low response rate for the staff survey is another limitation of the study, with response rates from staff in the L&D units varying from 15.8 percent to 98.2 percent. To the extent that there was self-selection by respondents, there may be bias in the survey results regarding changes over time in staff perceptions or knowledge. This concern is mitigated by findings that observed changes were in the expected direction (e.g., increased knowledge or perceptions of improved teamwork). For three of the L&D units, response rates for the first and second surveys were generally similar, thus increasing confidence in interpreting their results. Response rates dropped for the other two units, which weakens those findings. We have high confidence in the contents of the survey, which were obtained from existing, well-tested instruments.

Another limitation was our inability to do observation studies at both baseline and the end of the evaluation, also due to budget constraints, which prevented us from estimating teamwork performance changes over the study year based on independent observations of practices. For those observations conducted, the scores obtained represent a sample of practices at three shifts per site during one day of operation, which could have differed from practices on other days or times during the day. To mitigate this limitation, we developed scores for 12 one-hour data points during the observation periods, which could capture explicitly any variations in practices within those time periods.

In the outcome analysis, the low frequency of individual types of adverse events is a limitation that affects the ability to detect changes in outcomes. For this reason, we used the AOI in our analysis, rather than each of the ten individual types of events that comprise the AOI. This prevented us from examining more closely which types of adverse events might be affected most by teamwork improvements. Even using the AOI as the measure, the numbers of events were small enough that they varied visibly over time, thus reducing the power to detect changes in the measure for any individual L&D unit.

CHAPTER THREE

Findings Regarding Teamwork Implementation

This section presents the results of our process evaluation, which examines the participating L&D units' implementation of teamwork practices to achieve sustainable team-based care. These results address the first study objective—to better understand the conditions and actions required for hospital L&D units to achieve effective and sustainable teamwork practices—and its two associated research questions: What training and actions are required to achieve a high level of teamwork in the L&D process? And how strongly do self-reported experiences in implementing teamwork improvements correlate with actual levels of teamwork as measured by direct observation of the L&D process?

The sources of data for the process evaluation were the site visits conducted at the start of the study year, the monthly update calls with the implementation leads for each L&D unit, the final-assessment teleconference interview conducted at the end of the study year, and on-site observations of teamwork practices at each L&D unit at the end of the study. The initial site visit and bimonthly calls generated near-real-time data that yielded insights on the dynamics of the processes involved and efforts required to achieve strong, team-based care. The retrospective perspectives provided by the units in the final-assessment interviews identified multiple lessons that could benefit others embarking on similar teamwork-improvement implementation processes. The observational data helped us to calibrate and interpret our findings from the process evaluation.

Each L&D unit was one case study with its own unique organizational context, patient characteristics, and operational setting and methods. Using the process-evaluation data collected, we characterized the diversity of teamwork strategies and actions undertaken by the five L&D units, and we searched for common themes, issues, and lessons that cut across the experiences of all of them. The results presented in this chapter address three analytic goals:

- Characterize the nature and intensity of teamwork-practice implementation by each participating L&D for consideration in analysis with the outcome-analysis results to assess which factors are most important for successful implementation of teamwork practices and related effects on outcomes.
- Document the experiences, successes, challenges, and lessons learned for the participating L&D units in their implementation process.
- Provide sufficient information for five case examples on the processes and experiences of the participating sites, to help guide other L&D units in their own implementation activities.

Baseline Status and Teamwork Strategies Pursued

When conducting a study of this type, it is important to consider carefully the baseline status of each of the participating units regarding the practices being implemented and studied. Their initial status is the starting point from which the L&D units must move, and it therefore influences their strategies and approaches to implementation activities.

Site 1

This site is a large L&D unit in a community hospital that does not have a medical residency program. The unit had not acted to implement teamwork improvements until the start of this study. When it started work, however, it did so with a strong sense of urgency to achieve improved teamwork as quickly as possible because the hospital board of directors and executive management had made it a high priority and were pushing for fast action. Its basic approach was both structured and strongly proactive, working under the leadership of an interdisciplinary implementation team. The physician leader was actively engaged throughout the process, and the unit designated a separate physician champion with dedicated time for that role. It had a facilitator who coordinated and supported the team activities. Several months after starting implementation, it established an operations team that was given hands-on clinical responsibility to perform key coaching roles.

Site 2

This site is an academic medical center in an urban area, which is a referral center for other hospitals (many of them difficult-delivery cases). The unit had begun teamwork improvement in the year before this study started, but its momentum had eroded somewhat. It used this study to inject new energy into the work to further its progress. The hospital was committed to achieving effective teamwork and was pursuing it in other units of the hospital. The L&D unit took an approach of pursuing incremental progress by implementing subsets of teamwork practices over time, rather than working with many practices at once. A planning team guided the teamwork-improvement strategy and activities, with clinical coaching and implementation roles led by a separate coordinating team. The unit had a strong physician leader who directed much of the strategy, as well as a facilitator who coordinated and supported the team activities.

Site 3

This site is a large L&D unit in a suburban hospital with a medical residency program. Although it had been an intervention site in the original L&D teamwork study, the site had not implemented most of the teamwork practices. Its approach was to work on a variety of specific practices using a flexible strategy. The work was led by the obstetrics (OB) resource-management group, which oversaw the unit operation, including this teamwork initiative. This group subsequently became the Patient Safety Task Force. It also established the physician team leader program, which implemented a rotating position with each designated leader responsible for supervising team activities throughout the unit. The unit did not have a teamwork facilitator.

Site 4

This site is a large L&D unit in a regional referral center with a medical residency program. It had been an intervention site in the original L&D teamwork study, and it had already implemented many aspects of teamwork practices. As a result, it took an incremental approach to working with specific teamwork practices during the time covered by this study, focusing on refining and reinforcing them. The work was led by a team that was essentially the same group as the Maternal Child Executive Committee. It did not have a teamwork facilitator. It took an informal approach to coaching, using a one-on-one approach to coach during delivery of care.

Site 5

This site also is a large L&D unit in a regional referral center with a medical residency program. The unit had not acted to implement teamwork improvements until the start of this study. It took an incremental approach to working with specific teamwork practices, taking time to reinforce those being implemented at each time. The work was led by an interdisciplinary implementation team, which met relatively infrequently. Most of the implementation leadership was carried out by the physician leader and nursing leader. Using a train-the-trainer model for teamwork training, about 20 clinical personnel were trained to serve as trainers for others. The unit's approach for coaching staff was opportunistic reinforcement of skills during care processes.

Implementation Priorities and Actions

All of the participating L&D units started their work by organizing their implementation teams, which then designed and carried out their implementation approaches. The first actions they all took was to conduct initial training for staff working in the L&D units, using either the MedTeams or TeamSTEPPS training model. Following the training, they proceeded with implementing the practices or behaviors that are part of the teamwork model. Despite this apparent similarity in approach, the sites differed in how they carried out each of these steps. The specific approaches used by the sites for organizing their implementation teams, designing their initial training, and emphasizing each of the four basic teamwork competencies (early or later) in their implementation processes are summarized in Table 3.1.

Team Organization and Operation

As indicated in Table 3.1, the sites' implementation teams varied widely in terms of both size and manner of operation. One or two sites used large teams, whereas the others used teams with smaller membership. Sites 1 and 2 started with just an implementation team, which site 2 called a *planning team*. Each of them subsequently introduced another team that was responsible for the hands-on implementation of teamwork practices and coaching of staff in their use. For both sites, the implementation teams then limited their roles to guiding the overall implementation strategy and overseeing progress in carrying it out. As their operational teams became more active, the meeting frequency for their implementation teams declined, but they were able to maintain the engagement of team members and viable team activities.

Each of the other three sites worked with just one implementation team. In some cases, their teams were small right from the beginning; in other cases, the teams declined in numbers over time as work was focused in the hands of the team leaders. They all experienced difficulties in maintaining momentum for their teams, resulting in declines in the frequency of meetings over time.

Table 3.1
Basic Organization and Strategy for Teamwork Improvement of the Labor and Delivery Units

Site	Team Organization	Training of Staff	Competency Emphasis
1	Implementation team at start Added operation team Met regularly Had a facilitator	Initial TeamSTEPPS training for all staff in two months Additional training after seven months	Initial: leadership and communication Later: situation monitoring and mutual support
2	Large implementation team (planning team) Met regularly Coordinating team Had a facilitator	Initial MedTeams training for all staff over a six-month period Ongoing informal training	Initial: situation monitoring and communication Later: mutual support and leadership
3	Small implementation team; met periodically Had physician team leader program No facilitator	Initial TeamSTEPPS training for core leadership team in one session No formal training for others	Initial: leadership and communication Later: some emphasis on situation monitoring
4	Small implementation team Met periodically No facilitator	Initial TeamSTEPPS training for core leadership team in one session No formal training for others	Initial: situation monitoring and communication Later: leadership and mutual support
5	Large implementation team Met periodically No facilitator	Initial TeamSTEPPS training for core leadership team in one session No formal training for others	Initial: communications and mutual support Later: situation monitoring

Teamwork Training and Coaching

The sites differed in their training approaches, depending in part on whether they had been trained previously as part of the original study. In some cases, they had the full two-day TeamSTEPPS training; in others, they chose to use the shorter training module, depending on the staff audiences involved. What we focused on in the analysis was the extent of coverage of the training across the staff working in the L&D units—whether they trained all staff or just some of the staff. Regardless of training approach, the sites reported that the participating staff gave positive feedback about the training and were enthusiastic about the teamwork concepts and practices.

Sites 1 and 2 trained all the staff on their L&D units, although they used different approaches. Site 1 used an intensive schedule for initial training, through which it completed training for all its unit staff in two months, at the end of which it started activities to implement teamwork practices. Site 2 took six months to complete the training for all its staff, at the end of which it started activities to implement teamwork practices on the unit.

Sites 3 and 4 had done previous training as intervention sites in the earlier study. Both of these sites conducted initial training at the start of this study for only a subset of staff who had been identified to serve in lead roles in implementing teamwork practices on the units. Once trained, using a train-the-trainer model, these staff then were to train and coach other staff on the unit during teamwork practices implementation. For site 3, this training was required for any physician who took part in the team leader program. Site 5, which had not been an intervention site in the previous study, was the other site that trained only some of its unit staff.

Implementation of Teamwork Improvements

Implementation strategies designed and carried out by the five sites differed widely, both in the emphasis they place on the four teamwork model competencies and in the order in which they implemented the specific teamwork practices. The four teamwork competencies are leadership, situation awareness, mutual support, and communication (see Chapter One for description). As shown in Table 3.1, the sites took differing approaches in their choices of which competencies to emphasize initially versus later in their implementation process. However, all of the sites emphasized communication skills early in their implementation processes, seeing effective communication across clinical disciplines as an essential aspect of achieving strong teamwork.

The only specific practice for which all the sites took similar actions was the team huddle/brief, which they all introduced at the start of implementation. In these team huddles, all clinical staff meet to discuss cases at the change of shift from night to morning shifts. The sites' use of the huddles diverged somewhat over time. Some sites added regular team huddles at other changes of shift; some discontinued use of the morning huddles; some added spontaneous huddles to manage caseload challenges; and some added patient-specific huddles to manage care for individual patients on an as-needed basis.

For all the other teamwork practices, the sites varied widely in which of the practices they worked with first and which they deferred until later in the implementation process. Some sites introduced all of the practices at the start of implementation, after which they focused on just a few of them through coaching and reinforcement of staff behaviors. Others chose to start with a subset of the practices, and, after they made progress in implementing them, they then introduced other practices. The sites noted that they had the greatest difficulty implementing the debriefs and DESC script because they were not intuitive for staff. For example, some sites developed written guidance for staff on how to do debriefs, and they learned from practice how best to carry them out. Despite this difficulty, staff were very receptive to the use of debriefs as a real-time feedback mechanism from which they could learn, in some cases asking for a debrief after they had managed a particularly difficult case.

For ease of reference, Table 3.2 provides brief definitions of the teamwork practices (see Appendix A for more-detailed descriptions).

Achievement of Practice Adoption and Internalization

Given the variation in the pace at which sites introduced the teamwork practices, it is not surprising that they also varied in the time and extent to which they were able to internalize (fully implement) each practice so it became a normal part of "the way things are done here" in the L&D units. The schedules by which the five sites implemented each of the teamwork practices are presented in Table 3.3. In the table, "E" represents early internalization of a practice within the first four months of the study year, and "L" represents later internalization, after the fourth study month. "W" is used if the site was still working on internalizing a practice at the time the study ended.

All the sites reported that they internalized the team huddles/briefs early—the only practice addressed early by all of the sites. Some sites also internalized several other practices—situational awareness, SBAR, and hand-off techniques. Conversely, the practices that moved most slowly toward internalization were debriefs, the two-challenge rule, call-outs, and checkbacks. Several sites reported that they still were working on these practices at the end of our study, and some did not work on them at all (as shown by the empty cells in the table).

Table 3.2
Brief Definitions of Teamwork Practices

Practice	Description
Team huddle/brief	A meeting at which team members develop a shared understanding of the plan of care by discussing patients' status and sharing departmental information May be regularly scheduled or ad hoc
Debrief	A review of the management of a case to identify strengths and opportunities for improvement in performance Helps the team develop team skills and identify breakdowns in teamwork that affected patient care
Situational awareness	A tool to monitor situations, with a focus on STEP
Two-challenge rule	A specific strategy for providing spoken support, addressing conflict, and preventing errors in potentially ambiguous situations First challenge is in the form of a respectful question; second challenge includes provision of information to support the concern
DESC script	A strategy that may be used to manage all types of conflict May be especially useful in resolving affective conflict Steps include describing the situation, expressing one's feelings about it, suggesting alternatives and seeking treatment, and stating consequences in terms of their impact on performance goals
SBAR	A strategy that team members can use to communicate clearly and concisely The abbreviation denotes the types of information that should be communicated among physicians and other members of the health-care team: situation, background, assessment, and recommendation
Call-out	A technique used to provide information to all team members in a timely manner by announcing important or critical information to the whole team during emergencies and at other times requiring timely information
Check-backs	A strategy that addresses closed-loop communication to ensure that the receiver understands the information sent as the sender intended
Hand-off techniques	Techniques that enhance information exchange at critical times, such as shift changes and breaks, consisting of notifying team members of changes in coverage, conveying all necessary information to others, updating the patient-information board, and alerting the team that a hand-off has occurred

Site 1, which pursued a proactive implementation strategy, reported that it had internalized all the practices except the DESC script by the end of the study. It completed most of these later in its implementation timeline. Site 2 reported internalization of four practices, and it still was working on four others at the end of the study. These results may reflect its use of a gradual and persistent approach to implementation, which extended over a longer time period than did the strategy used by Site 1. Site 5 had mixed progress in achieving full implementation of the specific practices.

Sites 3 and 4 were intervention sites for the original study and had started implementation work before our study began. Both sites internalized several practices early in their timelines, but neither pursued a proactive implementation strategy during our study. Site 3 reported that it did not internalize any other practices, and Site 4 reported internalizing the two-challenge rule later in its timeline. Both still were working on the rest of the practices at the end of our study.

Table 3.3
Achievement of Teamwork-Practice Internalization Reported by the Labor and Delivery Units

Practice	Site 1	Site 2	Site 3	Site 4	Site 5
Team huddle/brief	E	E	E	E	E
Debrief	L	W	W	W	L
Situational awareness	E	L	E	E	
Two-challenge rule	L	L		L	W
DESC script	W			W	
SBAR	L	W		E	E
Call-out	L	L	W	W	W
Check-backs	L	W	W	W	W
Hand-off techniques	L	W	E	E	

NOTE: Data on achievement of internalization for each practice were self-reported by each L&D unit. The observation studies were done as an independent assessment of their status at the end of the study. E = early (first four study months). L = later (after month 4). W = working (still working on it at the end of the study). An empty cell indicates that that site did not work on that practice at all.

Implementation Experiences

As part of the monthly update teleconferences with the participating sites, we asked them to identify what their greatest successes and challenges had been since our previous call with them. This allowed us to track changes in their experiences over time as they worked on implementing teamwork practices in their L&D units and to identify factors that may commonly affect progress in teamwork implementation.

The successes the sites reported, which are summarized in Table 3.4, reveal the progress of their implementation activities during the year we tracked them. The key successes reported by each site are grouped by the first, second, and third portions of the total time we tracked them. The types of successes identified included those related to overall management of and response to teamwork improvements, as well as implementation of specific actions. The maturation of the organization and work of their implementation teams is reflected in the successes that several sites reported regarding effectiveness of their implementation teams and the growing receptivity of unit staff to teamwork practices. Sites 1 and 2, in particular, focused on their team operations and how they matured over time. All of the sites also identified a variety of successes in implementing specific actions during the course of our study.

Perhaps the strongest indicators of the sites' progress in implementing teamwork practices were the outcomes reported in the final third of the study, which suggested that their work was having effects on their care processes and patients. For example, Site 1 cited its success with a new protocol for emergency Cesarean sections (C-sections), and Site 2 cited a reduction in C-section infection rates. Site 3 cited improved customer satisfaction scores and its successful handling of an overload incident, through which it avoided adverse events. Site 4 reported that it had integrated teamwork principles and training into the unit activities and quality initia-

Table 3.4
Successes Reported by the Participating Labor and Delivery Units, by Time Period

L&D Unit	First Time Period	Second Time Period	Third Time Period
Site 1	Growing participation in team huddles/briefs, resulting in improved care coordination Growth in staff buy-in Clarification of team roles that gave new momentum to practice adoption Use of teamwork tools to deal with unanticipated events Reports by staff of how teamwork is helpful in managing events	Morning team huddles/briefs going well consistently, with good participation Less negativity by staff Creation of separate administrative and operations team structure, leading to highly functioning team structure Refresher session on SBAR by external consultant Improved quality of communication among physicians and nurses Staff internalizing the skills and talking about teamwork frequently	Morning huddle/brief very sustainable; one of the most important actions taken Increased physician buy-in Continued success of operations team Reinforcing behaviors and enthusiasm Fast staff response to emergency team huddles Central area where huddles/briefs held serving as an information hub Debriefs getting strong results in teamwork improvement Success with a new protocol for emergency C-sections Successful mock code called by NICU
Site 2	Better organized as a result of the coordinating team Professional growth in some staff, especially clerical staff Emergency response team has worked well Triage team effectiveness, especially for nurses and clerical staff	Implementation of the TPAC as an incentive program to use the practices Establishing the picture board of all staff on duty Implementing use of the triage phones Successful use of debriefing	Maintenance and commitment of planning committee Communication through individual meetings after debriefs and follow-up Better communication and interactions with NICU and pediatrics Staff development in teamwork skills Holding more debriefings with broad participation Reduction in C-section infection rates
Site 3	Good group initial training that created enthusiasm Staff embracing teamwork model with enthusiasm, despite implementation obstacles Getting the physician team leader program operational	Multidisciplinary teamwork between L&D, NICU, and anesthesia	Physician-nurse council is working well Staff willingness to take an active role in teamwork practices Improved customer-satisfaction scores Engagement of new nursing staff Successful handling of an overload incident, avoiding adverse events
Site 4	Implementation plan developed Provider acceptance of teamwork Maintaining priority on high level of teamwork, and no near misses or errors, despite staff shortages Good interdisciplinary collaboration	Good interdisciplinary communication between L&D and NICU A best-practice guideline for operational vaginal delivery that was very well received	Generating momentum with the nurses through additional training Change in the culture of the unit Integration of teamwork principles and training into the unit activities and quality initiatives (e.g., decreasing maternal lacerations)
Site 5	Improvement in communication due to team huddles/briefs at morning shift change	None reported	Debriefs have matured; now doing them for good events as well as bad events

NOTE: TPAC = teamwork-practice award card.

tives, which may be a reflection of the relative maturity of its teamwork activities at the start of the study.

The challenges reported by the sites are summarized in Table 3.5, which lists the challenges separately based on their origin from internal and external sources. This information shows that the sites faced challenges throughout their implementation activities and that the challenges tended to be similar across sites. Commonly reported internal challenges were incomplete training, inadequate coaching, staff resistance, slow uptake of new practices, erosion of implemented practices, and sustainability. The most commonly reported external challenges were construction, competing initiatives, staff shortages, leadership changes and support, and caseload increases. Although the challenges tended to change over time, some of them persisted for extended periods of time.

Retrospective Assessments by the Participating Labor and Delivery Units

In the final-assessment teleconferences held at the end of the study with each participating L&D unit, we asked the implementation leads to think back over their experiences in implementing teamwork improvements during the past year and to share with us what they learned during that process. In particular, we asked them to focus on feedback that would be useful to other organizations that are embarking on initiatives to strengthen their teamwork practices. We heard consistent themes from all the sites for many issues and factors, but their feedback also highlighted the diversity of approaches they used, reflecting the unique situation and organization of each individual site.

The Teamwork Implementation Team

Our inquiry into the implementation team included questions about how the sites designed and operated their teams, as well as the roles of physician champions and facilitators. We also asked them to discuss what they learned about managing the implementation process and any challenges they faced during this process.

The Importance, Role, and Activities of an Implementation Team. All of the sites highlighted the importance of having an active, multidisciplinary implementation team, but they took different approaches to their team functions. In particular, all the sites thought that the team was important in the early stages of an improvement initiative, to plan and guide the start-up of the teamwork implementation activities. Once the implementation is under way, their teams tended to function more in an oversight role and to meet less frequently over time. One site divided its initial implementation team into two groups—an administration team that provided the overall oversight and an operations team of front-line clinical staff that was "hands on" in carrying out the actions to implement new teamwork practices and coach staff on their use.

The sites emphasized that having representation from all the disciplines involved in L&D on the implementation team was important to get buy-in and ensure that their planned actions were feasible and actually carried out. The sizes of their teams ranged from eight to 20 people, with the larger teams generally used to ensure broad representation on the team. One site added support personnel to the team, such as environmental services, later, noting that it would have been wise to do that from the outset because they are an important part of the unit's team.

Table 3.5
Challenges Reported by the Participating Labor and Delivery Units, by Time Period

L&D Unit	First Time Period	Second Time Period	Third Time Period
Site 1	Internal: Hard to keep the momentum going Slow progress in getting everyone on the same wavelength External: Staff shortages for vacation schedules Competing initiatives using staff time Disruptions from construction Increased caseload and acuity Shortage of physicians because some have left the staff	Internal: Keeping up the momentum Rolling out SBAR and SWAT, which require more individual responsibility Providers' sense of vulnerability as their work becomes more transparent in a teamwork culture Difficulty engaging private-practice physicians in teamwork practices External: Unexpected nursing-staff shortages Gearing up for construction and renovation	Internal: Difficulty getting staff to do conflict resolution in real time rather than delay taking action Inability to do mock codes in the birthing unit as planned Need to reinforce the regular use of call-outs and check-backs Need to determine role of and establish an operations team External: Competition from other initiatives that lead to loss of momentum
Site 2	Internal: Problem getting buy-in from some staff, especially some in leadership roles Slow progress in empowering staff to speak up for patient safety Difficulty developing the core team concept with key teamwork practices Inability of many staff to address peers in conflict resolution using DESC script Getting staff commitment to mutual assistance and respectful communication as a standard for performance External: Stressed by an increased number of maternal transports to unit	Internal: Lost momentum of coordinating-team meetings and function of PSCs Need to tighten up triage team function Staff not remembering to carry and use the cell phones for triage Keeping teams and teamwork in place under the stress of crisis situations Other responsibilities make it hard for leaders to do active coaching External: Keeping the teamwork structure in place with an overwhelming workload Implementation of provider order entry, which has distracted staff	Internal: Trying to maintain the teamwork momentum and also get work done Difficulty in engaging individuals in teamwork who are unapproachable Slow progress in making teamwork part of the culture, requiring reinforcement External: Staff turnover resulting in new, less-experienced L&D staff Heavy workload
Site 3	Internal: Lack of coaching Lack of buy-in among some staff Inadequate training for nurses and residents External: Nurses spend time looking for supplies rather than providing care Nursing-staff shortages Other initiatives compete for staff time High census of high-acuity patients Facility renovations	Internal: Difficult to disseminate information throughout the OB unit Resource constraints restrict actions External: Other initiatives that compete for staff time and attention Changes in hospital policy Continued nursing-staff shortages	Internal: Resistance of some staff members, mostly on the night shift Inability to complete training for many staff due to lack of faculty to teach Difficult to keep new nurses engaged in teamwork practices External: None reported

Table 3.5—Continued

L&D Unit	First Time Period	Second Time Period	Third Time Period
Site 4	Internal: None reported External: Staffing shortages and turnovers Temporary move of L&D unit for renovations Temporary loss of a key physician lead Short staffed for physicians and nurses	Internal: Lack of teaching and coaching by the nurse trainers despite their enthusiasm after they were trained Some resistance from nurses External: Relocation back into original area, which might impair the level of teamwork achieved in the smaller temporary space	Internal: Reminding people to use the skills during physician leader's absence for two months External: Demands on their time from other initiatives that compete with teamwork
Site 5	Internal: Difficulty holding team meetings Lack of support from leadership chain External: Shortage and turnover of head nurses Changes in physician staffing and leadership	Internal: Continued lack of support from leadership chain External: New product-line directors less supportive of nurse practitioners	Internal: Lack of support from leadership chain Limited physician support Lack of participation by nurse midwives More training needed External: Change in physician leadership with less support by new leaders Staff turnover

NOTE: SWAT = strength, weakness, and threat analysis. PSC = patient service coordinator.

In general, the sites' implementation teams met weekly or biweekly at the start of their implementation processes, and the meeting frequency declined over time. They found that it was difficult to get everyone to the meetings due to competing time demands. They also found that having a consistent meeting time is important and that it is best to meet at a time when representatives from all shifts were able to participate.

All of the implementation teams used their meetings to strategize, review implementation progress, troubleshoot, and adjust implementation approaches. Some did this using structured team meetings with agendas, action plans, and timelines, while others used more-informal meeting formats.

One site noted that its team spent too much time early in the implementation process planning how to do it rather than just getting started. They realized they were "overthinking" things as they tried to define the roles and personnel of their administrative and operations teams. Once the team became more outcome-driven, it moved things along more quickly.

The implementation teams used a wide variety of methods for communication among team members and between the team and the front-line unit staff. For example, both email and face-to-face conversations were used for communication among team members. Methods used by one site to communicate with unit staff and get feedback from them included staff meetings, its patient-safety culture survey, safety rounds, shift reports, discussion in various venues, and observation on the unit.

Importance of Having a Physician Leader or Champion. The sites were unanimous in emphasizing how important it is to have a physician champion visibly leading teamwork-improvement efforts for the L&D units. They reported that a physician detractor can be very detrimental, and the physician leader can help other physicians overcome skepticism, as the message is more palatable coming from another physician. Having additional physicians teaching classes and role modeling also helps with buy-in.

The physician leader needs to be a driver who makes change happen and is visible at the key teamwork activities, such as daily morning reports (team huddles/briefs). The leader must be flexible and adaptive—not rigid—about the implementation. One site noted that the leader does not have to be someone who supported teamwork improvement from the outset.

Importance of Having a Designated Person to Facilitate the Implementation-Team Activities. Only two of the sites had facilitators who provided ongoing support for the implementation team and the teamwork activities they were implementing. Both facilitators were registered nurses, so they could relate effectively to the clinical staff. The role of their facilitators was to coordinate and support activities of the implementation team, provide data for decisions, perform outreach to clinical staff, analyze data on processes and outcomes, and generally help to move actions forward. These two sites reported that the facilitation role was an important stimulus for their continued progress in teamwork implementation. They said that it is important for the person serving as facilitator to have the time and interest to do the job well, to not have a clinical affiliation with the various groups, and to be able to work above the various silos in the organization.

The sites that did not have facilitators felt that such a person could have helped them increase progress in their implementation activities. One site reported that it had an effective educator on the team early in the process who contributed to their progress but that it lost that person in personnel changes. Resource constraints prevented the unit from hiring another person to serve in this role. To be most effective, the team leaders at this site said that the facilitator should report to someone in the unit so that his or her responsibilities are clear. Leaders at another site agreed that a facilitator sounded like a good idea, but they also felt that having clinicians model the teamwork behaviors is probably more helpful than having a facilitator involved.

Responding to Challenges That Arise During Teamwork Implementation. The sites reported that flexibility and perseverance are the most important factors for successful teamwork implementation. They emphasized the need to continually assess their implementation process to determine whether it was feasible and to make adjustments as necessary. An example reported by one site's team was its attempt to implement core teams, which it pursued unsuccessfully for some time. Then the team stepped back and realized that core teams were not necessary, given its implementation of some of the other practices, and that the concept was not feasible for that facility. If the team had been too dogmatic about pursuing the concept further, it could have lost credibility with the staff. Another site highlighted the importance of tracking outcomes to help focus the work. By identifying an issue (e.g., management of stat C-sections or codes) and then developing an organizational response, the unit could improve performance through tangible activities that contributed to teamwork development.

Teamwork Training and Coaching

To learn from sites' experiences with teamwork training, we examined three aspects of the training process: initial training on teamwork practices, ongoing coaching and reinforcement during implementation, and refresher training.

Best Approaches for Initial Training on the Teamwork Model and Practices. As described in the previous section, the sites took quite different approaches to the provision of teamwork training to their L&D unit staff. Two of the sites provided initial training to all the unit staff, although they differed in the pace at which the training was given. The others trained only a portion of the staff, then relied on the trained staff to train and coach the remaining staff in real time as teamwork practices were being implemented. Despite these differences, we heard very similar feedback from the sites regarding how the initial training should be designed and carried out.

The sites emphasized that the training should be interactive and that it should be multidisciplinary in terms of both the participants and the teachers. The use of interactive classes with videos and clinical scenarios specific to the unit made it realistic to the participants. Several of them found that it was effective to have medical doctors (MDs) and RNs teaching the sessions together. They also found that the environment and class size were important and that a class of about 15 participants was about the right size. One site specifically reported that use of the small-group approach was effective for them. Another site suggested that the training should be separate from the normal workday and include time for social interactions among participants.

Adequate time should be taken to develop the curriculum, to ensure the quality of the training provided. In addition, the curriculum should be modified to be relevant to the unit. Use of an outside consultant also was helpful, to provide expertise and an objective perspective. One site noted that it used the "parking-lot" method to record issues and concerns that participants raised so they could be addressed during later discussions. This proved to be invaluable because it assured people that their concerns were not being dismissed.

One site took six months to train all its staff, thus creating, for some staff, a delay between the time of their training and actual start of actions to implement the teamwork practices they were taught. As a result, the people who were trained early had forgotten the material when it came time to implement, and they needed reinforcement of their training at the start of implementation. The site team concluded that it might be better to condense the training to shorten this lag time.

Best Ways to Provide Ongoing Guidance to Unit Staff on Teamwork Practices. As the sites implemented teamwork improvements, they used a variety of techniques to reinforce and coach unit staff on use of effective teamwork practices. All of them reported that such reinforcement was critically important because they were working to change existing behaviors that were comfortable to staff, even if they were not optimal for effective teamwork. They noted that everyone must coach everyone, as "we are all learning as we go."

The use of coaches or coaching is central to the process of practice reinforcement. One site formally selected coaches early in the implementation process. The rest of them, however, relied on implementation-team members, lead physicians, and staff who had received teamwork training to take on this role, without officially designating them as coaches or providing them with designated time to perform this role. Some of the sites found that practice adoption flourished when the unit leaders modeled practices for others during care delivery. This shifting of the norm of behavior was a powerful way of influencing the reluctant individuals.

Leadership by physicians was an important component of the implementation process for all the sites. In some cases, it was the physician champion who reinforced practices; in other cases, one or more other physician leaders were designated to serve as coaches.

Careful selection of effective coaches is critical to achieving teamwork improvements. One site initially chose people who were less supportive in the hope that they would buy into the improvement process—a strategy that worked for only some of the coaches selected. Another site noted that its physician leaders varied in the quality of leadership they provided, with some being actively involved and others being more passive. The sites generally felt that they had not used coaches to the fullest extent needed, in part due to time and resource constraints. They felt that it would be ideal if coaches could be freed up from some of their other responsibilities, but few of them had the resources to do so.

Most-Effective Approaches for Conducting Refresher Teamwork Training. Because the final interviews with the sites were conducted within approximately a year after most of them had started their teamwork-improvement initiatives, few of them had much experience with providing refresher training. Therefore, their responses in this area were somewhat tentative.

Some sites said that they had not yet done any formal refresher training, but they had provided regular reinforcement in daily reminders, daily team huddles/briefs, staff meetings, debriefings, morbidity and mortality conferences, and other settings. They were not sure how effective these various methods had been, and they considered this to be a work in progress. One site questioned whether there was a need at this time for a refresher for existing staff because the teamwork behaviors were becoming so ingrained for them. Others believed there would be value to having a shorter refresher course to revisit the behaviors and contemplate whether they are doing all they could.

On the other hand, most of the sites had established teamwork training as part of the orientation training for new employees and staff. One site also provides training for new physicians, which appeared to be working well.

Implementing Teamwork Improvements

Success or failure in implementing teamwork improvements can be affected by a myriad of factors, including how the implementers choose to carry out the process, as well as external factors that may reinforce or challenge their ability to do so. We discuss here the feedback from the sites regarding their implementation activities and what they learned from their experiences with them. This is followed by discussion of some of the environmental factors that the sites identified as having affected their implementation progress.

Which of the Four Teamwork Competencies to Work on First. The four basic competencies of the MedTeams and TeamSTEPPS models are leadership, situation monitoring, mutual support, and communications. Our inquiry into the sites' strategies for addressing each of these competencies revealed broad differences in the priorities the sites placed on each competency. For example, the two sites that were most proactive in implementing changes differed in which competencies they chose to address first. One of the sites started by working on leadership through team huddles/briefs and establishing the team structure. Its team felt that this needed to be done before it could move on to the other competencies. The other site put leadership at the bottom because, even if one of the leaders is opposed to an idea, the group can work around him or her. The other sites tended to see leadership as an important competency that they worked on early.

The sites were in greater agreement on the importance of the communication competency, and all of them addressed communication early. One site started its training curriculum with communication, and it used team leaders to facilitate and model the behaviors. Another site saw communication as critical to situation monitoring and mutual support, by empowering people to question and challenge others in a respectful way. Communication skills also are concrete skills that staff can learn readily.

The sites agreed on the importance of situation monitoring and mutual support, but they again differed on when they focused on practices in these competencies. One site felt that situation monitoring and mutual support should go hand in hand. According to this site,

> If you are monitoring the situation, you are more likely to offer support. Initially, physicians were resistant to the concept of situation monitoring due to liability concerns, but it is now a nonissue. We now have the philosophy that everyone is responsible for everyone's patients.

Other sites focused on each of these two competencies separately, with an apparent emphasis on situation monitoring. One site noted that it was useful to start with situation monitoring to help break the historical approach that "this is my patient and nothing else matters." Another site emphasized that situation monitoring is critical to patient safety (i.e., monitoring for staff fatigue) and is not a "big brother" situation, nor is it judgmental.

Which of the Specific Teamwork Practices to Introduce First. In addition to the four basic teamwork competencies, the MedTeams and TeamSTEPPS models specify a set of specific teamwork practices or behaviors that staff are to use during the care process. We were interested in learning how the sites approached introducing these specific practices and how their choices for use of the practices affected their progress in teamwork improvement.

The sites felt that all practices should be adopted eventually but that they could be prioritized and phased in over time. The sites also had quite different approaches to deciding the order in which they introduced each practice. Their priorities for the implementation plan generally were drawn from discussions in the initial training sessions, and the sites also used the training materials for guidance.

Most of the sites started by introducing the team huddle/brief, although they used a variety of names for them (e.g., team report, board rounds). The units typically used these sessions to set the initial care plans for the shift, and they encouraged all members to participate. They noted that the huddle can be used to change the flow of activities on the unit, and huddles around specific patients also are done when care planning cannot be deferred to the next team huddle.

Some of the practices (e.g., hand-offs, SBAR) are being advocated by the Joint Commission, which makes them a natural choice for early introduction. Several sites saw that SBAR could be used for case presentations at team huddles, though few had done this by the end of this study.

Debriefs and DESC script were identified as important practices that are hard to do well. One site team felt that debriefs give the biggest bang for the buck but were the hardest for them to "get off the ground." Another site developed a tool to guide the discussion quickly, and the leaders worked to be sure that everyone recognized that the debrief was a learning process, not a punitive one. Because of the difficulty in using the DESC script, the units struggled with using it, and at least one unit decided not to use it.

One site decided to implement all the specific practices at once but found that team huddles/briefs, situational monitoring, and debriefs have been the most-important tools for the unit. They said that they started with practices that are more mechanical and gave them the opportunity to demonstrate some early success, after which they moved to the more-abstract and emotionally charged issues. Sites reported that one-on-one coaching was required to get many of the practices implemented properly.

Approach to Engaging the Key Clinical Groups in Teamwork Improvement. All of the sites faced challenges early in their implementation processes in encouraging physicians and nurses to support and participate in the teamwork methods they were introducing. In general, although they met some initial resistance from at least some of their staff, reactions to the idea of improving teamwork tended to be positive. In addition, staff support increased over time as teamwork improvements began to show benefits in the efficiency and quality of care. However, the sites emphasized that it was important to work with the unit staff to ensure that they were given the opportunity to participate and influence the actions being taken to introduce and implement teamwork practices.

The following are examples of techniques that the sites felt were successful in engaging physicians and nurses in the teamwork-improvement process:

- Role modeling was done by leaders among both physicians and nurses, which was found to be critically important.
- Several sites found that team huddles/briefs (morning rounds) have been key to engagement with physicians and nurses together.
- Teamwork behaviors and success stories were featured regularly with posters, mentions in daily team huddles/briefs, and other communication vehicles.
- During clinical education with physicians, they talked about teamwork tools and not just diagnosis; teamwork education should be part of any clinical education.
- Teamwork-practice sessions also were used as a basis for other meetings and gatherings to strengthen a sense of team and partnership among staff.
- At one site, all staff saw the Josie King video.
- At one site, nurses reviewed some aspect of teamwork at each shift change.

The sites also offered the following guidance on important issues or steps to take:

- Leaders need to stress that effective teamwork is important because these are evidence-based practices to improve patient care.
- It may take time (estimated three to six months) for unit staff to see how teamwork practices improve patient care, after which increased engagement builds among staff.
- For one site, high nursing turnover made it challenging to ensure that nurses on the unit were adequately trained in teamwork practices.
- Teamwork is a dignified process designed to formalize best practices, so it is not necessary to use gimmicks and T-shirts to encourage engagement.
- Observed success in implementing teamwork in one unit can spread it to others. At one site, people working on the maternity unit could see the differences in the quality of care processes between their unit and the birthing unit (which implemented teamwork), and they became anxious to get on board.
- Each unit should adapt the approach to naming and implementing the teamwork model to make it "belong" to the unit, to instill a sense of ownership for the unit staff.

Most-Important Mechanisms Implemented to Improve Teamwork. Consistent with other feedback provided by the five sites, the mechanisms they reported being most important were the start-of-shift team huddles/briefs (board rounds), physician leadership and coaching, administrative support through the implementation process, QI meetings, and debrief. Debriefings were viewed as an opportunity to evaluate care and learn how to strengthen the use of teamwork practices.

The team huddles are a strong mechanism for getting everyone on the same page for a shift, and they encourage communication across disciplines. At some sites, these sessions were introduced first at the morning change of shift, and then staff on later shifts requested the same approach. One site, however, discontinued these sessions in favor of smaller interactions throughout the day, which encourage staff to be mindful of the practices in all day-to-day encounters.

Importance of Continually Reinforcing New Teamwork Practices. All the sites had worked throughout the year of the study to reinforce new practices, and they all stressed that such perseverance was necessary to achieve sustainable teamwork practices on their units. One site commented that shifting the norm of behavior is a powerful way of influencing reluctant individuals. Another noted that some strategies worked well in the short term, but it shifted to other methods for the long term. The use of debriefs was cited as a strong tool, not only to improve care as part of teamwork practices, but also to reinforce the learning of those practices.

They all highlighted the importance of ongoing coaching to help staff learn in real time, recognizing that everyone must be coaching one another, as they were all learning as they progressed. However, the sites took very different approaches to the coaching process. For example, one site started with charge nurses as coaches but later turned to its implementation team to do the coaching. Another site used designated physicians as coaches. Regular reinforcement and celebrating of successes also were important strategies, such as featuring success stories in communication activities.

What They Would Do Differently

In hindsight, the sites identified things they would do differently in the various aspects of the implementation process: planning, training, carrying out actions, coaching, and creating incentives for teamwork behaviors. They saw the importance of good planning by the implementation team but also said that they could have moved into action more quickly. One site reported that its tendency to "overthink" issues and strategies delayed its start for actually making change happen. The sites also said that they would establish more-realistic timelines for their action strategies, recognizing that it takes time to change human behavior. Some of the sites that did not have facilitators indicated that they would want to have one, although budget constraints made that impossible during this implementation process. Some sites also noted that other incentives are needed to encourage staff to adopt team practices, such as including team behaviors in personnel evaluations.

The sites that did not do initial training for all their staff said that it was better to train everyone quickly, to get them all on the same page. Similarly, most of the sites commented that they would place stronger emphasis on coaching, including formal designation of coaches so that all the staff knew that the coaches were available to work with them. For both training and coaching, however, the sites were constrained by resource limitations that prevented them from supporting the activities in the way they thought was optimal.

Factors Affecting Teamwork Implementation

We asked the sites to identify the factors that had the greatest effect on their ability to implement teamwork improvements, either positively or negatively. We specifically asked them to consider both process factors involved with the implementation process itself and other factors that were external to the process (whether in the hospital or in the larger environment).

Process Factors. The implementation of any QI process is inevitably affected by issues that arise in response to the implementation activities. When we asked the site leads to identify the most-important factors that affected their teamwork implementation processes, they reported the following items:

- initial hesitancy or resistance from physicians and other staff, which generally declined as experience showed that improved teamwork was positive for the staff delivering care on the units. Some of the initial physician resistance was due to liability concerns.
- continued resistance from a small number of nurses and physicians, often those who were long-term employees, which was reported by most of the sites. Although the resisters were a small percentage of the staff, they could have a big effect on the unit operation. In some cases, this played out in the departure of some physicians or nurses, and several of the teams also were considering actions to terminate some resistant staff.
- the need for strong support for the teamwork-improvement work from the top hospital administrative leadership, which includes the visible presence of leaders at training and other key activities, as well as dogged support and encouragement from leaders as the work progressed
- designing the training to be multidisciplinary, such that physicians and nurses are taught together in all training sessions, and sessions are co-taught by physicians and nurses
- resource constraints for some sites that limited the amount of training and implementation actions that they could undertake

- heavy workloads and turnover for physicians and nurses in the units that tended to constrain the extent of implementation actions that some sites could carry out
- heavy daily volumes of L&D patients that had the positive effect of stimulating use of teamwork practices. Some sites reported that they achieved a great deal of collaboration on very busy days, and team members learned that improved collaboration and teamwork can help the unit deal more effectively with workload issues. For example, their use of cross-monitoring, mutual assistance, coaching by the coordinating team, and negotiation between staff and providers through impromptu huddles improved dramatically during the very busy times. However, this began to occur only after they had been working for some time on implementing teamwork practices.
- a positive impact of staff turnover on implementation, reported by one site, with newer staff being more receptive to new practices than some of the long-term staff who left
- the ability to build a sense of team spirit among all the staff in the unit, which was necessary to reinforce their ability to work together in adopting the teamwork practices
- changes in health information technology that were stimulated by requests from staff for more information to enhance situational awareness
- use of communication technology, such as pagers and cell phone, to achieve greater real-time communication among front-line staff, although limitations of the various technologies and inconsistency in staff use of them diminished their usefulness.

External Factors. The units' responses to external factors affecting their progress mirrored the set of successes and challenges reported in Table 3.4 and Table 3.5, so we do not repeat them here. However, two issues emerged that merit specific attention: insurer support and the physical layout of the L&D units.

One site identified insurer support as a positive factor. The insurer encouraged the hospital to implement teamwork, as well as other patient-safety practices, including a review of oxytocin use, use of standardized protocols, an exam for electronic fetal monitoring, and lowering surgical-site infection for C-sections. The insurer supported these efforts by funding a safety nurse for OB in all hospitals participating in its initiative. This person served as this site's team facilitator, which the site team felt was an extremely important contributor to their progress in teamwork implementation.

The units' physical structure had a variety of influences on their teamwork implementation activities and progress. For one unit, physical barriers in the unit configuration drove its need to strengthen communication across sections. As a result, the unit staff now have better awareness of what is going on in the different areas, including OR and triage. The unit configuration for another site hampered its triage process. One site reported that the physical environment impeded its attempts to implement core teams because its unit has just one corridor that does not provide separate sections for multiple teams. Another site reported that renovations in the hospital forced the unit to move locations twice, which posed a challenge for implementing and sustaining teamwork improvements.

Ideal Physical Environment to Support Effective Teamwork Practices. Given the issues raised about the physical layout of the units, we specifically asked the sites to identify what they thought would be an ideal physical environment to support effective teamwork. Because L&D units have widely varying physical floor plans, hospital layouts, and equipment setups, responses to this question about ideal physical environment are equally varied. The following observations are reported here as examples of how the physical environment can influence the process and results of implementing improved teamwork in any given unit.

- Private space is needed for conducting debriefs.
- A large centralized location is needed for conducting change-of-shift team huddles.
- Patient-care pods create a physical separation that makes it very difficult to increase teamwork unless the unit can staff around this configuration.
- A single, central work area should be provided for physicians and nurses, with smaller satellites near the patients for smaller groups to meet.
- A separate triage area would be helpful.
- A smaller unit area supports cross-monitoring and mutual assistance.
- Registration should be configured so that a clinician is available to the patient immediately.

Concluding Questions

We concluded the final-assessment interview with the site teams by asking them to share what they thought were the greatest successes, challenges, and surprises experienced during their teamwork implementation processes. Finally, we asked what advice they would give to other L&D units that are about to embark on similar journeys.

Greatest Successes Thus Far in Achieving Effective Teamwork. When asked what their greatest successes were, several sites cited improvements in communication that allowed them to talk about what was best for the patient, including more-respectful communication among staff. They also said that they increased overall collaboration and mutual assistance on the unit, such as staff volunteering to contribute to processes, which had not occurred previously.

Improvement in teamwork culture was also a strong theme in the sites' responses. One site reported that teamwork has become such a part of its culture that everyone looks at how it is relevant to any given situation. Another reported a decreased stress level on the unit due to greater interdisciplinary camaraderie and openness, with much less reluctance to ask questions of physicians and raise issues. Yet another said that its staff were doing well in crisis situations, indicating that a good foundation had been laid.

Greatest Frustrations or Disappointments. The inability to get all the unit staff on board with teamwork was disappointing to most of the sites, which referenced a small number of individuals in their units who remained resistant to the change. In some cases, these holdouts were leaders on the unit, and they influenced the tone of the group when they were present at meetings. One unit expressed frustration at not being able to figure out how to convince them of the need for change or demonstrate to them that they were not acting appropriately.

Other disappointments mentioned were lack of progress in using the DESC script and limitations in coaching success. Those reporting these issues also noted that they were continuing to work on them, which reflects their recognition that teamwork was still a work in progress for their units.

Biggest Surprises from Actual Teamwork-Improvement Experience. The most common response by the sites regarding their biggest surprises was their very success in improving teamwork. The sites observed growth in the staff as a result of using the teamwork practices, and they reported that they could see their progress clearly by comparing their resulting unit operation to that of other units in the hospitals. One site team thought that its success might be due in part to infusion of new staff who were receptive to the concepts. One site was surprised by the success of the debriefing, which had stimulated open communication between nurses and physicians.

Overall Advice to Other L&D Units to Enhance Their Success in Improving Teamwork. We concluded the interview by asking the sites to offer advice to others based on their experiences in teamwork implementation. They provided the following suggestions:

- Examine teamwork status at the outset. For example, identify which practices the unit might already be using and which need to be strengthened.
- Present team-based care to the staff in training so that it is palatable, then reinforce the training. Without reinforcement, most staff forgot the practices on which they had been trained. One site chose to introduce the material in smaller segments to make it more palatable.
- Train enough trainers so that the practices are reinforced and coached routinely by a number of people.
- Repeat emphasis and training on use of practices to reinforce them and educate new staff.
- The implementation process takes a long time and should not be rushed. A good strategy is to start with practices that staff can see clearly will improve patient care, then add the other less-concrete practices later.
- Commitment from nursing leadership and educators is essential for reaching the staff.
- Incorporate teamwork practices into personnel evaluations.
- Do periodic check-backs to assess progress and impacts. The sites reported that the teleconferences and discussions that were part of this study helped them with this.
- Measure progress and give feedback to staff regularly. One way to do this is with patient-safety culture surveys. One site that used a survey saw improvement in staff perceptions of teamwork over time.
- In private hospitals, administration has limited influence on attending physicians.
- Achieving sustainable teamwork will take more time and resources than one might expect.
- Do not get frustrated when progress is not apparent. Persistence is critical. It is worth doing—one must have a "Zen-like" approach to avoid frustration.

Observed Teamwork Practices

The observation studies we performed at the participating sites at the end of the study enabled us to compare the self-reported information the sites provided us in the site visits and teleconference interviews to an independent, expert observer's assessment of their teamwork performance. The results of the observation studies, presented in Table 3.6, are sets of average scores for each site on each of the four competencies of teamwork practices—leadership, situation monitoring, mutual support, and communication—plus the structural dimension of team structure. Scores reported are overall average scores (and standard deviations) for each teamwork aspect for the full 12 hours of observation, as well as average scores for each of the three four-hour components of the total observation time. The scoring used a five-point scale (where 1 = very poor and 5 = excellent).

We found variation in observation scores across sites, across time periods within a site, and across teamwork competencies within a site. The highest-performing site overall was site 4, which was scored at 4.5 or higher for all five teamwork aspects and had consistent performance

Table 3.6
Results for Observations of Actual Teamwork Practices, by Site

Teamwork Competency	Overall Scores		Means by Time Period		
	Mean	Standard Deviation	Period 1 Evening	Period 2 Evening/Night	Period 3 Night/Day
Site 1					
Team structure	3.3	0.1	3.3	3.2	3.3
Leadership	4.0	0.0	4.0	4.0	4.0
Situation monitoring	3.9	0.1	3.8	4.0	4.0
Mutual support	3.8	0.4	3.6	3.8	4.1
Communication	3.3	0.5	3.3	3.0	3.6
Site 2					
Team structure	3.7	1.4	2.1	4.8	4.3
Leadership	4.0	1.5	2.2	5.0	4.8
Situation monitoring	3.9	0.9	2.9	4.4	4.4
Mutual support	4.1	1.0	3.1	4.9	4.4
Communication	4.0	1.0	2.8	4.6	4.8
Site 3					
Team structure	2.8	1.2	4.0	1.8	2.5
Leadership	3.0	1.2	4.3	2.2	2.6
Situation monitoring	2.4	0.8	3.3	1.7	2.1
Mutual support	2.8	1.4	4.3	2.2	2.0
Communication	3.1	0.8	3.8	2.9	2.6
Site 4					
Team structure	4.6	0.6	4.3	5.0	4.3
Leadership	4.5	0.3	4.2	4.8	4.6
Situation monitoring	4.5	0.3	4.3	4.8	4.3
Mutual support	4.5	0.4	4.1	4.8	4.6
Communication	4.6	0.1	4.6	4.6	4.7
Site 5					
Team structure	3.9	0.4	3.7	4.0	4.0
Leadership	3.9	0.4	3.6	4.3	3.9
Situation monitoring	3.4	0.5	3.0	3.5	3.8
Mutual support	3.9	0.3	3.8	4.3	3.7
Communication	3.8	0.3	3.6	4.0	3.7

NOTE: Scores are on a five-point scale: 1 = very poor and 5 = excellent.

across time periods. Sites 1, 2, and 5 also had reasonably high scores. The scores for sites 1 and 2 varied across teamwork aspects, reflecting differences in the timing by which they had focused on each competency in their implementation strategies. Sites 2 and 3 appeared to have the greatest variation in teamwork practices across shifts, as reflected in the standard deviations of the overall scores, which suggests that their progress in implementing practices differed by shift.

To examine the extent to which the sites had strengthened their teamwork practices, we used a combination of the qualitative, self-reported interview data and the observation data presented in Table 3.6. Because we did not have baseline observation data (due to budget constraints), we could not directly examine changes in observed practices from baseline to the end of the study. When comparing the observation results to the self-reported information, both the baseline levels and changes in practices over time needed to be considered. For example, site 1 had done no previous work on teamwork before this study, but its implementation team took a proactive and organized approach that was successful in implementing a substantial number of teamwork practices during the year. The observation scores for site 1 reflected respectable teamwork practices at the end of the study, but they were not scored as high as site 2 or site 4, both of which had started teamwork implementation before the time of this study.

Site 2 leaders had been using an incremental, gradual approach to implementation, which continued during this study. Although its observation scores were high, they varied across shift and, somewhat, across teamwork aspect. These results are consistent with its implementation history. The site 4 leaders consistently reported in our interviews that they were already doing many of the practices in the teamwork model and that they used the model primarily to reinforce these practices for their staff. We also heard this feedback from their staff during the site visit. This information is consistent with the high observation scores given to site 4.

By contrast, sites 1 and 5 were just starting their work at the start of this study, so they did not have teamwork practices in place at our baseline. Site 1 took a structured and organized approach to implementing a teamwork-improvement strategy, whereas site 5 focused more directly on implementing specific practices using an operational approach. They had similarly high observation scores, although the scores for site 1 varied more across teamwork aspects. Again, these results also are consistent with its implementation history.

Site 3 had been an intervention site in the previous clinical trial study, but it reported that, after its staff received the training in that study, it had not pursued any teamwork improvements at that time. Thus, it also was starting these activities as our study began. However, the site experienced several challenges and setbacks in both the teamwork implementation activities and challenges imposed on it from external sources, which prevented it from making much progress in practice adoption. Site 3 had the lowest performance observation scores, which appear to be confirmed by the observation data as well.

We would expect that the teamwork performance of the two sites that already had implemented some teamwork improvements before our study began would change less during the study than would performance of other sites that started during the study and pursued actions proactively. Their performance at our baseline would be higher than the other sites, which would provide them with less room to make additional improvements. Because site 2 continued its incremental and gradual approach to implementation during the study, we might expect to see some improvement related to this work. Site 4 took a more passive approach to its improvement efforts, which suggests that we might not see much improvement in teamwork. We examine this question further in our outcome analysis of the staff survey results and patient outcomes.

Key Process-Evaluation Findings

The results of the process evaluation highlighted the diversity of approaches that the L&D units chose for implementation actions aimed to achieve adoption of teamwork practices, and suggest that there is not one "correct" strategy for achieving adoption of the teamwork competencies or specific practices in L&D units. We summarize here what we learned regarding each of the research questions addressed by the process evaluation.

What Training and Actions Are Required to Achieve a High Level of Teamwork in the Labor and Delivery Process?

The key factors required for successful implementation the five participating L&D units appeared to be early emphasis on the communication competency of the teamwork model, along with effective training and coaching, support of a facilitator to keep the process on track, and unit-staff perseverance in working toward practice adoption. The other three teamwork competencies—leadership, situation monitoring, and mutual support—also were important to achieve, and they could be addressed successfully using a variety of approaches. For choices regarding introduction of the specific teamwork practices, the team huddle/brief was an important practice to adopt early in the implementation process, but the remaining practices could be addressed in the order that each unit found to be most appropriate.

The sites found the team huddle/brief to be a powerful tool that could provide a structure and stimulus for interdisciplinary communication, which could also create a sense of team among physicians and nurses. The morning team huddle was a strong vehicle to support morning change of shift and to ready the staff team for managing the day's patient caseload. In addition, the huddle was used both for emergency situations and for patient-specific care assessment and planning.

During the course of their work, the sites came to recognize the importance of providing initial teamwork training for all staff. Several of the sites did initial training for only some of their staff because of budget limitations or other operational choices. All of these sites stated that this led to slower staff buy-in and delays in adoption of teamwork practices. The sites reported substantial difficulties in getting staff trained later using coaching or informal training.

Perseverance was found to be key because it took time to fully integrate effective teamwork practices into L&D units, and challenges were faced throughout the implementation process. Even with a highly proactive implementation approach, these results suggest that it takes longer than a year to fully integrate effective teamwork practices into a unit's care processes. The two sites that had been working longest on implementation had the highest performance scores, whereas sites with only one year of implementation experience still had more work to do, even though some of them had made substantial progress. At the end of our study, the leaders of the teams for all of the participating L&D units reported that, although they had made important progress, their work was still not done.

Challenges may come from external sources or may be internal in the form of responses to the implementation efforts themselves. Typical challenges the sites experienced from external sources included staff shortages, construction projects, and competing initiatives. A common internal challenge was some initial staff resistance to teamwork improvement. Resistance tended to decline with time, however, as staff gained experience with teamwork and began to see its benefit in improving care and operational efficiency. Tension between physicians and nurses also occurred in the early implementation period, which the sites used as an opportunity to reinforce effective communication and mutual support skills.

How Strongly Do Self-Reported Experiences in Implementing Teamwork Improvements Correlate with Actual Levels of Teamwork as Measured by Direct Observation of the Labor and Delivery Process?

We found that the observation scores for teamwork performance varied across sites, across time periods within site, and across teamwork aspects within site. In general, the levels and variations in teamwork scores for each site were consistent with its self-reported implementation status as of the end of the study. For example, the leaders for site 4 reported that they had already been doing many of the teamwork practices before the start of the study, but they were generally passive in subsequent implementation work during the study. The high observation performance scores for that site were consistent with this information. If we had baseline observation data for this site, we would expect it to be high as well—that is, it would reflect the site's already-strong teamwork practices at baseline for this study.

Summary

These results highlight the fact that organizations could gain value from using observational studies to track implementation progress as they work on improving teamwork practices. Observations done by an external expert could provide them with objective data to identify issues and guide subsequent implementation actions.

The process evaluation found some common themes in the approaches used by the participating L&D units for implementing improvements to their teamwork practices, although their specific strategies and actions varied substantially. This information should be useful for other L&D units pursuing teamwork improvements, to guide them in ensuring fidelity to the teamwork models they choose to use while adapting strategies to their unique situations. The implementation actions that we identified as possibly being important contributors to achieving improved teamwork were initial training of all staff, follow-up coaching, support of a facilitator, and implementation of a large number of the specific teamwork practices. If these factors are important, their use should influence staff perceptions of teamwork in the L&D units, as well as patient outcomes, which we test in Chapter Four as part of our outcome evaluation.

Effects of Teamwork Improvement on Unit Staff and Patient Outcomes

This chapter presents the results of our outcome evaluation, which examined the effects that teamwork improvements made by the participating L&D units had on both the staff working in the units and the patients served by them. These results address the second study objective—to assess the extent to which successful adoption of teamwork practices may influence the experiences of staff working in the units and outcomes for patients—and its two associated research questions: How does achieving effective teamwork affect the patient-safety perceptions, experiences, and knowledge of staff working in L&D units? And what effects does effective teamwork have on L&D outcomes for mothers and newborn infants?

As discussed in Chapter Two, data for effects on unit staff were obtained from a survey conducted with the staff twice during the study. Data for effects on patient outcomes were obtained from encounter data that the L&D units provided to NPIC for analysis, the results of which NPIC provided to RAND.

Perceptions and Knowledge of Labor and Delivery Unit Staff

The first component of our outcome evaluation was an analysis of trends in patient outcomes for the participating L&D units. These analyses were performed to address the third research question for the evaluation: *How does achieving effective teamwork affect the patient-safety perceptions, experiences, and knowledge of staff working in labor and delivery units?*

To analyze effects on unit staff, we compared results from waves 1 and 2 of the staff surveys that were completed by staff working in the L&D units. These surveys provided data on the perceptions of L&D unit staff regarding patient safety and teamwork, the quality of their work lives, and their knowledge of teamwork practices.

In these analyses, we tested our hypotheses that teamwork improvements in the L&D units should have the greatest effects on staff perceptions about teamwork in the unit, the quality of their work lives, and staff knowledge of teamwork practices. Improvements might also affect staff perceptions of patient-safety culture in the unit and, to a lesser extent, perceptions of patient-safety culture at the hospital level. As discussed in Chapter Two, response rates for the surveys varied across sites and time, and they tended to be low; therefore, we interpret our findings with some caution.

Because we were analyzing survey results for two cross-sectional samples of staff, we checked for comparability of the respondent characteristics for the two samples. The results of this comparison, presented in Table 4.1, show fairly similar distributions for the two groups of respondents for time worked in the hospitals, time worked in this unit, staff position in the

Table 4.1
Respondent Characteristics in the Two Waves of Staff Surveys, Across All Sites

Respondent Characteristic		Wave 1		Wave 2	
		Number	Percentage	Number	Percentage
Time worked in this hospital (p = 0.884)	<1 year	47	10.4	27	11.2
	1–5 years	153	33.7	77	32.0
	6–10 years	96	21.2	50	20.8
	11–15 years	50	11.0	23	9.5
	16–20 years	42	9.3	24	9.6
	21 years or more	58	12.8	32	13.3
	Missing	8	1.8	8	3.3
Time worked in this hospital unit (p = 0.516)	<1 year	65	14.3	35	14.5
	1–5 years	158	34.8	75	31.1
	6–10 years	95	20.9	53	22.0
	11–15 years	51	11.2	19	7.9
	16–20 years	37	8.2	26	10.8
	21 years or more	37	8.2	24	10.0
	Missing	11	2.4	9	3.7
Job status in the hospital (p = 0.003)	Full time	303	66.7	179	74.3
	Part time	102	22.5	28	11.6
	Agency staff	2	0.4	0	0.0
	Contract staff	16	3.5	7	2.9
	Missing	31	6.8	27	11.2
Staff position in this hospital (p = 0.707)	Physician	131	29.5	73	30.3
	Nurse	216	47.6	113	46.9
	Other	96	21.2	46	19.1
	Missing	11	2.4	9	3.7
Time worked in current specialty or profession (p = 0.278)	<1 year	22	4.9	16	6.4
	1–5 years	111	24.5	66	27.4
	6–10 years	79	17.4	31	12.9
	11–15 years	71	15.6	28	11.6
	16–20 years	65	14.3	40	16.6
	21 years or more	98	21.6	52	21.6
	Missing	8	1.8	8	3.3

hospital, and time worked in current specialty or profession. The one area of difference was job status in the hospital, for which respondents indicated whether they were full-time, part-time, contract, or agency staff. Greater percentages of the respondents in the second survey wave were full-time staff than in the first wave, and there also was a higher percentage of data missing on this item for those who completed the survey.

Status at Baseline

We examined variations across the five L&D units in the baseline perceptions and knowledge of staff in the units. We grouped the domains for which data were obtained into five categories: hospital-level culture of patient safety, patient-safety culture in L&D, teamwork in L&D, quality of work life, and knowledge of teamwork. As shown in Table 4.2, significant variations in staff perceptions and knowledge across the sites were found and were statistically significant for all of the domains.

Two of the sites (sites 2 and 4) had systematically higher scores on the various domains than the remaining three sites (high scores shown in shaded cells). (The scores are measured as the percentage that gave scores of 4 or 5 on a five-point scale; see methods in Chapter Two). These two sites are the ones that already had been implementing teamwork practices before this study began, and this result is consistent with their reported implementation status at baseline.

We also found differences in scores across the domains. Respondents across the sites tended to give higher scores to hospital management support for patient safety, organizational learning/continuous improvement, and teamwork within the unit, and they gave lower scores for hospital hand-offs and transitions and nonpunitive response to error. Of interest, the patient-safety grades the staff gave their L&D units varied widely across units, ranging from 32.9 percent to 70.8 percent positive grades.

Changes in Staff Perception and Knowledge During Teamwork Implementation

Differences in staff perceptions and knowledge regarding teamwork between the baseline (wave 1) and second (wave 2) surveys were examined for all the sites in the aggregate and for each site individually. The larger sample size for the aggregated data provides more power to detect statistically significant differences that may not be detectable for individual sites. As discussed in Chapter Three, however, the teamwork implementation experiences of the five sites varied widely, and we might expect similar variation in the effects they had on the perceptions and teamwork knowledge of the staff in each site. Such differences are hidden in the aggregate results averaged across all five sites, so it is important to look at both the aggregate and individual site results when interpreting our findings.

The results of the aggregate analysis are presented in Table 4.3. For all domains except organizational learning, the percentages of respondents giving positive scores were higher for the wave 2 survey, although differences were statistically significant for only six perception domains and the knowledge-of-teamwork domain. The positive change in teamwork knowledge suggests that the combination of initial training and reinforcement during teamwork implementation increased staff knowledge regarding teamwork principles and practices.

The strongest changes were found for all three domains in the teamwork-in-L&D category, in particular for the domain of teamwork climate (from 56.3 percent to 65.4 percent). Significant changes also were found for two of the four domains in the culture-of-patient-safety-in-L&D category, and the domain of nonpunitive response to error had a large change (from 18.1 percent to 28.8 percent). The only significant change in the hospital-level-culture-

Table 4.2
Patient-Safety Attitudes and Knowledge at Baseline, by Site

Domain (n)	Site 1 (221)		Site 2 (72)		Site 3 (86)		Site 4 (32)		Site 5 (43)		p-Value
	%	SD	%	SD	%	SD	%	SD	%	SD	
Hospital-level culture of patient safety											
Hospital management support for patient safety	61.2	30.2	62.5	30.6	46.5	32.5	70.8	32.5	56.6	33.0	<0.001
Hospital hand-offs and transitions	27.0	40.1	44.4	44.8	23.3	37.3	43.8	45.3	11.6	28.5	<0.001
Organizational learning, continuous improvement	75.0	29.3	75.5	31.6	64.3	34.6	82.3	26.8	64.3	35.2	0.008
Teamwork across hospital units (one question)[a]	51.4	50.1	72.2	45.1	41.7	49.6	68.8	47.1	32.6	47.4	<0.001
Patient-safety culture in L&D											
Patient-safety grade	70.8	45.6	59.7	49.4	32.9	47.3	75.0	44.0	40.5	49.8	<0.001
Nonpunitive response to error	8.1	20.0	35.2	37.7	18.6	31.6	42.7	39.9	18.3	27.7	<0.001
Overall safety status in the unit	47.3	34.7	52.0	31.8	26.1	30.7	58.6	32.1	36.5	31.3	<0.001
Patient-safety climate in the unit	59.9	32.3	74.1	29.2	56.5	30.7	79.4	23.5	63.6	31.2	<0.001
Teamwork in L&D											
Teamwork within the unit	80.2	30.0	65.8	36.7	65.8	37.2	85.9	26.9	50.0	40.8	<0.001
Communication openness	43.1	27.6	55.4	22.5	48.6	24.4	58.9	18.4	45.0	26.1	<0.001
Teamwork climate	58.2	38.0	60.6	39.6	47.6	40.8	78.1	35.8	41.9	37.7	<0.001
Quality of work life	69.5	26.3	66.4	26.9	55.8	27.0	75.5	22.0	64.2	29.5	<0.001
Knowledge of teamwork[b]	67.7	19.8	70.3	20.0	61.8	17.8	71.5	17.7	69.8	17.3	0.025

NOTE: n = number of completed surveys. % columns indicate percentage that gave ratings of 4 or 5 on five-point scale (except knowledge domain). SD columns indicate standard deviation. Shaded cells contain the two high scores for each domain.

[a] Item was "Hospital units work well together to provide the best care for patients."

[b] Percentage of patient-safety knowledge questions answered correctly (out of eight).

Table 4.3
Changes in Patient-Safety Attitudes and Knowledge Across All Sites

Domain (n)	Wave 1 (454)		Wave 2 (241)		
	%	SD	%	SD	p-Value
Hospital-level culture of patient safety					
Hospital management support for patient safety	58.9	31.7	60.6	32.9	0.508
Hospital hand-offs and transitions	28.8	40.8	34.4	43.5	0.091
Organizational learning, continuous improvement	72.6	31.5	71.6	34.2	0.719
Teamwork across hospital units (one question)[a]	52.3	50.0	60.1	49.1	0.052
Culture of patient safety in L&D					
Patient-safety grade	58.8	49.3	63.8	48.2	0.223
Nonpunitive response to error	18.1	30.6	28.8	35.5	<0.001
Overall patient-safety status in the unit	43.7	34.3	49.7	35.5	0.033
Patient-safety climate in the unit	63.3	31.6	66.9	32.0	0.164
Teamwork in L&D					
Teamwork within hospital unit	72.4	35.0	78.7	33.1	0.022
Communication openness	47.6	25.9	53.0	25.7	0.010
Teamwork climate	56.3	39.4	65.4	37.7	0.004
Quality of work life	66.3	27.1	70.1	27.6	0.083
Knowledge of teamwork[b]	67.5	19.3	71.4	19.4	0.010

NOTE: n = number of completed surveys. % columns indicate percentage that gave ratings of 4 or 5 on five-point scale (except knowledge domain). SD columns indicate standard deviation. Shaded cells indicate statistically significant differences.

[a] Item was "Hospital units work well together to provide the best care for patients."

[b] Percentage of patient-safety knowledge questions answered correctly (out of eight).

of-patient-safety category was for the domain of teamwork across hospital units. These results are consistent with our hypotheses that the teamwork implementation activities would have their strongest effects on staff perceptions regarding climate and practices within the unit, rather than across the hospital as a whole. The quality of work life reported by L&D unit staff increased from 66.3 percent to 70.1 percent, but this difference was only marginally significant statistically (p < 0.083).

In Tables 4.4 through 4.8, the same results are presented individually for each of the five L&D units participating in the study. Reflecting their varied implementation processes and experiences, their staff survey results differ for many of the domains examined. Fewer significant changes were found for the individual sites than in the aggregate results. For four of the sites, no changes were found for any of the domains in the categories of hospital-level culture of patient safety or the culture of patient safety in L&D. Site 5 had one significant change in each of these categories, which were large increases in scores for the domains of hospital hand-offs and transitions and nonpunitive response to error.

Table 4.4
Changes in Patient-Safety Attitudes and Knowledge, Site 1

Area of Change (n)	Wave 1 (221)		Wave 2 (49)		p-Value
	%	SD	%	SD	
Hospital-level culture of patient safety					
Hospital management support for patient safety	61.2	30.2	58.5	35.7	0.580
Hospital hand-offs and transitions	27.0	40.1	29.6	43.2	0.692
Organizational learning, continuous improvement	75.0	29.3	74.1	29.9	0.849
Teamwork across hospital units (one question)	51.4	50.1	50.0	50.5	0.865
Culture of patient safety in L&D					
Patient-safety grade (one question)	70.8	45.6	73.8	44.5	0.698
Nonpunitive response to error	8.1	20.0	12.5	27.2	0.298
Overall patient-safety status in the unit	47.3	34.7	52.6	30.6	0.332
Patient-safety climate in the unit	59.9	32.3	67.1	31.6	0.166
Teamwork in L&D					
Teamwork within the unit	80.2	30.0	87.3	22.0	0.065
Communication openness	43.1	27.6	53.8	28.8	0.018
Teamwork climate	58.1	38.0	71.9	32.5	0.022
Quality of work life	69.5	26.3	70.0	27.8	0.901
Knowledge of teamwork[a]	67.7	19.8	76.3	14.5	<0.001

NOTE: n = number of completed surveys. % columns indicate percentage that gave ratings of 4 or 5 on five-point scale (except knowledge domain). SD columns indicate standard deviation. Shaded cells indicate statistically significant differences.

[a] Percentage of patient-safety knowledge questions answered correctly (out of eight).

The L&D unit staff at site 1 perceived improvements in two domains in the category of teamwork in the unit: communication openness and teamwork climate (both significant). This was the only site for which increases were found in this category. Perceptions regarding quality of work life increased only for site 2, and staff knowledge of teamwork increased for site 1 and site 3. All of these domains are within-unit measures, which we hypothesized would be more likely to be affected by teamwork-improvement activities than hospital-level measures would be. For the hospital-level measures, we found no significant changes in perceptions of the L&D unit staff at the individual site level.

Site 1 undertook a highly focused and proactive implementation process for teamwork improvement, as discussed in Chapter Three, and the survey results of perceived improvements for three domains are consistent with that effort. The other site that was actively implementing teamwork was site 2, for which we found a significant increase only for the domain of quality of work life. Because this site had started these activities almost a year before our study started, changes in staff experiences might have occurred before our wave 1 survey, which

Table 4.5
Changes in Patient-Safety Attitudes and Knowledge, Site 2

Area of Change (n)	Wave 1 (72)		Wave 2 (75)		
	%	SD	%	SD	p-Value
Hospital-level culture of patient safety					
Hospital management support for patient safety	62.5	30.6	64.4	35.7	0.724
Hospital hand-offs and transitions	44.4	44.8	44.7	44.7	0.976
Organizational learning, continuous improvement	75.5	31.6	74.7	36.3	0.888
Teamwork across hospital units (one question)	72.2	45.1	70.3	46.0	0.796
Culture of patient safety in L&D					
Patient-safety grade (one question)	59.7	49.4	70.6	45.9	0.187
Nonpunitive response to error	35.2	37.7	42.0	36.4	0.270
Overall patient-safety status in the unit	52.0	31.8	59.7	33.6	0.159
Patient-safety climate in the unit	74.1	29.2	72.3	33.4	0.727
Teamwork in L&D					
Teamwork within the unit	65.8	36.7	74.7	37.1	0.151
Communication openness	55.4	22.5	54.7	23.7	0.848
Teamwork climate	60.6	39.6	65.3	36.7	0.451
Quality of work life	66.4	26.9	75.5	26.5	0.042
Knowledge of teamwork[a]	70.3	20.0	69.5	20.2	0.806

NOTE: n = number of completed surveys. % columns indicate percentage that gave ratings of 4 or 5 on five-point scale (except knowledge domain). SD columns indicate standard deviation. Shaded cells indicate statistically significant differences.

[a] Percentage of patient-safety knowledge questions answered correctly (out of eight).

could not be captured by these two surveys. We consider this issue further in our conclusions in Chapter Five.

Although all of the other three sites had undertaken some teamwork-improvement activities, including initial training and various strategies to implement improved teamwork practices, their levels of activity during our study year were less focused and comprehensive than those of site 1 and site 2. Their more-limited approaches may be reflected in the few significant improvements in scores found in their staff survey results. Site 3 had an improvement only in knowledge of teamwork, with no significant increases in staff perceptions of patient safety or teamwork. No significant increases were found for site 4, and scores for some of its domains declined (although the declines were not statistically significant). On the other hand, site 5 had large increases in scores for the domains of hospital hand-offs and transitions, nonpunitive response to error, and teamwork within the unit, suggesting that the teamwork-improvement activities they undertook may have contributed to improved perceptions by their staff.

Table 4.6
Changes in Patient-Safety Attitudes and Knowledge, Site 3

Area of Change (n)	Wave 1 (86)		Wave 2 (55)		
	%	SD	%	SD	p-Value
Hospital-level culture of patient safety					
Hospital management support for patient safety	46.5	32.5	53.3	29.1	0.208
Hospital hand-offs and transitions	23.3	37.3	17.3	35.0	0.343
Organizational learning, continuous improvement	64.3	34.6	66.7	35.7	0.701
Teamwork across hospital units (one question)	41.7	49.6	48.1	50.4	0.458
Culture of patient safety in L&D					
Patient-safety grade (one question)	32.9	47.3	43.5	50.1	0.241
Nonpunitive response to error	18.6	31.6	13.3	25.3	0.299
Overall patient-safety status in the unit	26.1	30.7	28.2	35.4	0.704
Patient-safety climate in the unit	56.5	30.7	53.3	33.6	0.563
Teamwork in L&D					
Teamwork within the unit	65.8	37.2	65.7	38.6	0.995
Communication openness	48.6	24.4	47.5	26.4	0.796
Teamwork climate	47.6	40.8	47.2	40.9	0.947
Quality of work life	55.8	27.0	57.1	25.9	0.781
Knowledge of teamwork[a]	61.8	17.8	68.6	20.1	0.036

NOTE: n = number of completed surveys. % columns indicate percentage that gave ratings of 4 or 5 on five-point scale (except knowledge domain). SD columns indicate standard deviation. Shaded cells indicate statistically significant differences.

[a] Percentage of patient-safety knowledge questions answered correctly (out of eight).

Effects of Implementation Actions on Staff Perceptions and Knowledge

To examine possible effects of the sites' teamwork implementation actions on staff perceptions and knowledge, we estimated a series of logistic regression models in each of which the dependent variable was one of the domains covered by the staff survey (measured as 1 if the respondent rated the domain 4 or 5, or 0 if rated it lower). We hypothesized that the implementation actions would have the greatest effect on staff perceptions of teamwork within the L&D units, their quality of work life, and teamwork knowledge.

The process-evaluation results identified several implementation actions that might be most likely to lead to teamwork improvements and, therefore, to changes in staff perceptions, quality of work life, and knowledge. These actions were the implementation of teamwork practices, provision of coaching for staff, having a facilitator to support the implementation team, and the extent of staff training. The first variable was defined as "implemented more than three teamwork practices," the second was "provided coaching," and the third was "had a facilitator and trained all staff." We combined the facilitator and staff training actions into one vari-

Table 4.7
Changes in Patient-Safety Attitudes and Knowledge, Site 4

Area of Change (n)	Wave 1 (32)		Wave 2 (43)		
	%	SD	%	SD	p-Value
Hospital-level culture of patient safety					
Hospital management support for patient safety	70.8	32.5	60.5	31.9	0.172
Hospital hand-offs and transitions	43.8	45.3	36.0	0.7	0.454
Organizational learning, continuous improvement	82.3	26.8	68.2	33.3	0.053
Teamwork across hospital units (one question)	68.8	47.1	69.8	46.5	0.926
Culture of patient safety in L&D					
Patient-safety grade (one question)	75.0	44.0	64.1	40.6	0.330
Nonpunitive response to error	42.7	39.9	34.9	37.1	0.384
Overall patient-safety status in the unit	58.6	32.1	55.2	32.5	0.657
Patient-safety climate in the unit	79.4	23.5	73.0	27.6	0.298
Teamwork in L&D					
Teamwork within the unit	85.9	26.9	93.5	18.4	0.180
Communication openness	58.9	18.4	54.0	23.2	0.332
Teamwork climate	78.1	35.8	85.7	25.4	0.312
Quality of work life	75.5	22.0	73.7	26.3	0.757
Knowledge of teamwork[a]	71.5	17.7	72.4	20.5	0.840

NOTE: n = number of completed surveys. % columns indicate percentage that gave ratings of 4 or 5 on five-point scale (except knowledge domain). SD columns indicate standard deviation.

[a] Percentage of patient-safety knowledge questions answered correctly (out of eight).

able because those sites that had a facilitator also trained all staff, and the remaining sites did neither.

We created three dummy variables for these actions, for use as predictor variables in the regression models. Each was coded as 1 for wave 2 respondents if the unit in which the respondents worked had taken the relevant actions; otherwise, it was coded 0. All variables were coded 0 for respondents to the wave 1 survey (baseline), thus creating an interaction between survey wave and each action variable.

We estimated four logistic regression models. In the first model, we included independent variables for survey wave 2 and dummy variables for each of the sites. We added staff characteristics to the second model, and we then added interaction terms for site by survey wave to the third model. In the fourth model, we used the three training action variables and removed the site-survey wave interactions because using both sets of variables overidentified the model, requiring some to be dropped.

Presented in Table 4.9 is a summary of the regression results for five of the survey domains—teamwork in the L&D units, communication openness in the units, teamwork

Table 4.8
Changes in Patient-Safety Attitudes and Knowledge, Site 5

Area of Change (n)	Wave 1 (43)		Wave 2 (19)		
	%	SD	%	SD	p-Value
Hospital-level culture of patient safety					
Hospital management support for patient safety	56.6	33.0	71.9	22.9	0.071
Hospital hand-offs and transitions	11.6	28.5	52.6	48.5	0.002
Organizational learning, continuous improvement	64.3	35.2	75.4	34.9	0.256
Teamwork across hospital units (one question)	32.6	47.4	57.9	50.7	0.062
Culture of patient safety in L&D					
Patient-safety grade (one question)	40.5	49.8	66.7	48.5	0.071
Nonpunitive response to error	18.3	27.7	49.1	39.1	<0.001
Overall patient-safety status in the unit	36.5	31.3	51.3	38.6	0.117
Patient-safety climate in the unit	63.6	31.2	70.5	21.5	0.384
Teamwork in L&D					
Teamwork within the unit	50.0	40.8	77.6	32.2	0.011
Communication openness	45.0	26.1	57.9	29.1	0.088
Teamwork climate	41.9	37.7	55.3	43.8	0.224
Quality of work life	64.2	29.5	77.9	29.4	0.096
Knowledge of teamwork[a]	69.8	17.3	72.4	18.9	0.598

NOTE: n = number of completed surveys. % columns indicate percentage that gave ratings of 4 or 5 on five-point scale (except knowledge domain). SD columns indicate standard deviation. Shaded cells indicate statistically significant differences.

[a] Percentage of patient-safety knowledge questions answered correctly (out of eight).

climate in the units, quality of work life, and knowledge of teamwork (see Chapter Two for details on specification of these variables). (See Appendix G for detailed results of the regression models.) We summarize these briefly here, noting significant changes by site and by each of the teamwork action variables (with significant change defined as statistical significance of p ≤ 0.05).

The results shown in Table 4.9 indicate that all but one of the sites had significant improvements for *teamwork in the L&D units*. Only site 3 showed deterioration. However, none of the three teamwork action variables had significant effects for this domain (see model 4 in Appendix G).

We also found mixed performance among the sites for *communication openness in the units*, with some sites having significantly improved performance and others going in the negative direction. Two of the teamwork action variables—coaching and facilitator/training—had significant positive effects for this domain, while teamwork-practice implementation had a negative effect.

Table 4.9
Summary of Regression Results for Staff Perceptions and Teamwork Knowledge

Result Area	Significant Changes from Study Baseline to Study End[a]				
	Teamwork in the L&D Unit	Communication Openness in L&D Unit	Teamwork Climate in the L&D Unit	Staff Quality of Work Life	Staff Knowledge of Teamwork
Study site					
Site 1	Increase*	Increase***	Increase**	Increase**	Increase***
Site 2	Increase***	None	Increase***	Increase***	Decrease**
Site 3	Decrease*	Decrease***	Decrease**	None	Increase***
Site 4	Increase**	Decrease**	Increase*	None	Increase***
Site 5	Increase***	Increase***	Increase***	Increase***	None
Implementation actions					
More than 3 teamwork practices	None	Decrease*	None	None	Decrease**
Coaching provided	None	Increase***	Increase**	Decrease***	Increase***
Facilitator and trained all staff	None	Increase***	Increase***	None	Increase***

NOTE: * p < 0.05. ** p < 0.01. *** p < 0.001.

[a] Percentage that gave ratings of 4 or 5 on a five-point scale (except knowledge domain).

Four sites had improved performance on *teamwork climate in the units*, but site 3 had a decline in performance. Both the coaching and facilitator/training variables had positive effects on this domain; practice implementation had no effect.

Mixed results are found for effects on the *quality of work life* for staff. Three sites had improvements for this domain, while sites 3 and 4 had declines. None of the teamwork action variables showed positive effects; indeed, coaching had a negative effect on the domain.

Finally, *knowledge of teamwork* increased for staff in all the units except site 2, which showed a decline in knowledge. Both coaching and facilitator/training had positive effects on knowledge, but practice implementation had a negative effect.

These regression results are markedly different from those for the individual L&D units, presented in Table 4.4 through Table 4.8, reflecting the greater statistical power available with the regression models that used all the data for the five sites together. Statistically significant changes in staff perceptions for several domains are found for all of the sites. However, site 1 is the only L&D unit for which staff perceptions improved for all five domains considered. Site 5 had staff-perception improvements for four of the domains, and we found mixed results for sites 2 and 4. Site 3 improved on only one domain (teamwork knowledge) while its staff perceptions declined for three of the domains and did not change for one.

We also estimated effects for the other survey domains, but we do not present them here because they were either hospital-wide or more-general patient-safety measures, which are less directly related to the units' teamwork implementation actions. We did find improvements for more than one unit for overall patient safety, nonpunitive response to error, hospital management support for patient safety, teamwork across units, and patient-safety climate. In general, however, these effects were less consistent across sites than those for the domains on which we are focusing.

Effects of Teamwork Improvement on Patient Outcomes

The second component of our outcome evaluation was an analysis of trends in patient outcomes for the participating L&D units. These analyses were performed to address the fourth research question for the evaluation: What effects does effective teamwork have on L&D outcomes for mothers and newborn infants?

We used the ten patient-outcome measures developed in the original L&D teamwork trial, which include six measures of maternal outcomes and four measures of newborn outcomes. In addition, we examined trends in the two AOIs developed based on these measures (Mann et al., 2006). The AOI is a rate defined as the number of deliveries that had one or more of the ten specific outcomes, divided by the total number of deliveries. The WAOS is defined as the sum of the adverse-outcome scores of all specific outcomes, divided by the total number of deliveries, in which the score for each specific outcome is a weight that represents the relative severity of that outcome.

As described in Chapter Two, NPIC estimated rates for each hospital for each individual measure, the AOI, and the WAOS. NPIC calculated hospital-level rates on a quarterly basis for the calendar years 2005 through 2007, using encounter data provided by the sites. We used these data for our outcome analysis.

We established time-specific threshold points for each hospital to separate the baseline and implementation time periods, which were anchored on their dates of initial training. Anchoring the trend data for each site on the quarter in which it started implementing teamwork improvements, we plotted trends in the AOI and WAOS for the five sites. The AOI trends are shown in Figure 4.1, and the WAOS trends are shown in Figure 4.2.

If a site improved patient outcomes, the improvement would be observed on the graphs as a downward deflection in AOI or WAOS rates for quarters following the first quarter (Q1) of the implementation period, relative to its existing trend during the site's prestudy period.

Only the outcome trend for site 2 shows a change that suggests an effect that might be related to the site's teamwork improvements. This site had a baseline trend of increasing AOI rates, followed by declining rates during the implementation period, which suggests some improvement in patient outcomes that might be related to the site's implementation activities. The trends for the remaining sites do not reveal such improvements in either the AOI or WAOS rates. The AOI rates for site 1 moved downward slightly during baseline and appeared to continue declining during the implementation period (Figure 4.1). Site 4 had a steadily declining trend in AOI rates from baseline through the implementation period, suggesting that their implementation actions may not have altered its baseline trend. Trends for site 5 show no change in AOI rates over time.

We encountered problems in the data provided by site 3, such that its AOI and WAOS trends abruptly dropped almost in half during the implementation period. We verified with NPIC that the data for NICU admissions were the source of the problem, which NPIC was not able to resolve with the site. Therefore, we do not report these data here, nor did we include them in our regression analyses.

Figure 4.1
Quarterly Trends for Adverse Outcome Index for the Five Sites

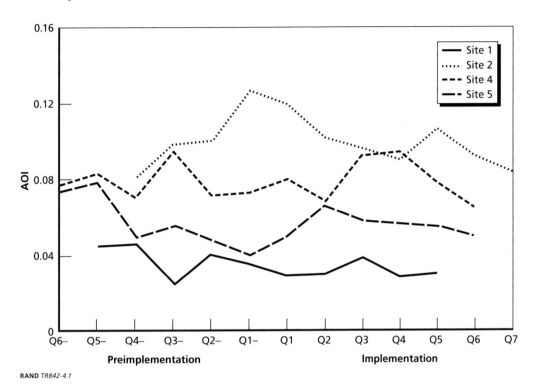

Figure 4.2
Quarterly Trends for Weighted Adverse-Outcome Scores for the Five Sites

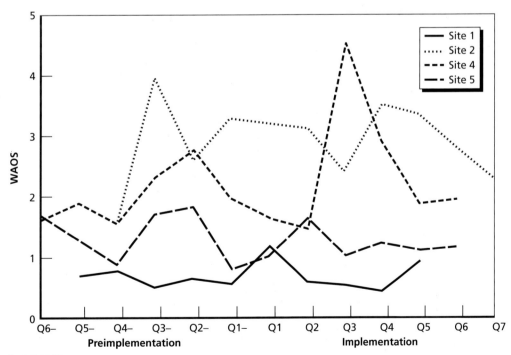

As described in Chapter Two, to test the relationship between AOI scores and teamwork training and implementation done by each site, we estimated a grouped logistic regression for each site separately. We used a piecewise linear function for time with a single knot (i.e., two linear segments) denoting the quarter in which the teamwork training took place, using two formulations that allowed us to assess whether AOI outcomes changed, as well as what effect the training itself might have had on any identified changes:

1. The quarter in which teamwork training was implemented was included in the second segment (i.e., the teamwork training quarter was included in the post period under the assumption that its effect would be immediate).
2. The quarter in which teamwork training was implemented was included in the first segment (i.e., the teamwork training quarter was included in the pre period under the assumption that its effect would not be immediate).

The regression results, shown in Table 4.10, confirm what is observed in Figure 4.1, finding a significant change in trend only for site 2. Further, the change is slightly more significant for formulation 1, in which the training is included in the implementation period, suggesting that training has an effect as part of the intervention.

Site 1 exhibited a significant decline in AOI over time, but the implementation of teamwork training did not significantly affect the rate of decline. Site 4 did not exhibit a significant change in AOI over time associated with teamwork training using either formulation. Site 5 did not exhibit a significant change in AOI over time associated with teamwork training using either formulation.

When the outcomes for site 2 are weighted by severity (the WAOS rates), however, these trends disappear. The WAOS rates for site 2, shown in Figure 4.2, fluctuate up and down over time. Looking at the WAOS rates alone, site 2 may be seen as not having affected occurrence of adverse events during deliveries. Combined with the (possibly) decreasing AOI rates, it is possible that site 2 reduced some adverse events but that the events that did occur were those with more-severe effects on patients (i.e., with larger WAOS weights).

Similar changes to trends occurred for the other three sites with usable trend data, resulting in generally flat trends in WAOS rates. In fact, the WAOS rate for site 4 spiked in Q3 of the implementation period, suggesting that one or more unusually severe events occurred during that quarter. Its rates subsequently dropped back down to previous levels.

Table 4.10
Results of Logistic Regressions That Tested Trend Changes in Adverse-Outcome Index, by Site

Site	1. Training in Implementation Period	2. Training in Baseline Period
Site 1	Not significant	Not significant
Site 2	p = 0.02	p = 0.06
Site 4	Not significant	Not significant
Site 5	Not significant	Not significant

Key Outcome-Evaluation Findings

The results of the outcome evaluation suggest that the teamwork implementation efforts of the L&D units participating in the study influenced staff experiences in working in these units, but outcome effects for reduction in adverse events for mothers and newborns were found only for site 2. We view effects on staff experiences to be proximal effects that are likely to occur within a short time following the start of an intervention—in this case, teamwork implementation. Effects on maternal and newborn outcomes are more-distal effects that might take a year or more to be observable after the start of implementation of teamwork improvements. We summarize here what we learned regarding each of the research questions addressed by the outcome evaluation.

How Does Achieving Effective Teamwork Affect the Perceptions and Experiences of Staff Working in Labor and Delivery Units?

The improvements in staff experiences were observed as differences in staff responses to two surveys conducted about eight months apart. We found improvements in staff perceptions of teamwork, especially for domains closest to teamwork in the L&D units—teamwork practices, communication openness, and teamwork climate—as well as for quality of work life and teamwork knowledge. However, the sites varied with respect to domains for which staff perceptions improved, ranging from improvements for all five domains for site 1 to improvement in only one domain for site 3.

We also found significant relationships between improvements in L&D unit-staff perceptions and two of the three measures for implementation actions—coaching and initial training/facilitator support during the teamwork implementation process. However, the effects of these implementation actions varied across the domains of staff perceptions. Staff perceptions did not appear to be affected by how many of the specific teamwork practices had actually been implemented by the units. These results suggest that successful adoption of a large number of the specific teamwork practices may not be an important factor in changing staff perceptions and knowledge of teamwork in the L&D units.

What Effects Does Effective Teamwork Have on Labor and Delivery Outcomes for Mothers and Newborn Infants?

Only site 2 had an observable and significant effect on maternal and newborn outcomes, which was a decline in its AOI rates during the teamwork implementation period. Its WAOS trend did not change, however; nor did we find changes in the WAOS trends for the other sites. The results for site 2 suggest that site 2 might have reduced the frequency of less-severe events but not total overall severity on patients. This interpretation was given support experientially by the lead of this site, who reported that the site does continue to experience infrequent high-severity events, even though overall frequency of events has declined.

These generally null findings may reflect the nature of the outcome measures used. Most of them are very low-frequency adverse events, for which stable trends are difficult to establish, as we documented in a recent study of teamwork outcome measures (Sorbero et al., 2008).

It also is possible that one year is not long enough for improved teamwork to become sufficiently integrated into a unit's health-care processes to produce observable effects on patient-outcome measures based on adverse events. Teamwork improvements might have affected other aspects of patients' experience with their OB care that are not captured in these measures. For example, data from patient surveys might reveal that implementation of teamwork practices was associated with improvements in patients' satisfaction with care.

Summary

The outcome evaluation found variations across sites regarding changes in staff perceptions on teamwork, quality of work life, and knowledge, and it found limited improvements in patient outcomes. These findings tended to be consistent with what we learned in the process evaluation regarding which sites made the most progress, and at what speed, in adoption of sustainable team-based care.

CHAPTER FIVE

Synthesis of Findings and Conclusions

The purpose of this study was to improve understanding of what is required to achieve effective and sustainable teamwork practices and improvements in related outcomes. The study results have given us a substantial portion of the answer to that question, although some uncertainties remain. From the process evaluation, we have learned that a diversity of approaches to implementing teamwork improvements can be successful but that any of these approaches should include several actions that appear to be keys to progress. The L&D units that successfully implemented the largest number of teamwork practices were those that provided comprehensive initial training to all staff working in the L&D unit, followed that training with one-on-one coaching throughout the implementation process, emphasized effective communication as a core teamwork competency, had a facilitator who supported the implementation process, and persevered in efforts to achieve improved teamwork practices.

These process-evaluation results were reinforced with outcome-evaluation results that showed improvements for several of the participating L&D units in both teamwork knowledge for staff working in the units and their assessments of teamwork climate and practices in the units. These improvements also were found to be associated with having a facilitator and training all staff, as well as with use of ongoing coaching. At the same time, we found effects on maternal and newborn adverse outcomes for only one site (site 2), despite our expectation that at least some improvement in outcomes might be observable within a year following the start of teamwork implementation.

Synthesis of Findings from the Study

Through this longitudinal study, we have been able to develop rich information about the complex processes and dynamics involved in implementing improvements to teamwork practices, through which L&D units have striven to achieve effective team-based care. We witnessed the units modifying their strategies and actions over time as they learned from experience and their initiatives matured, and they progressively implemented a growing number of specific teamwork practices. Because we captured their status on a monthly basis, we did not have to rely on their memories of earlier experiences or issues, which would have risked introducing recall bias. The study has revealed the complexities of these processes, which required major cultural changes within the L&D units to achieve these results and cannot be done quickly.

We were not surprised by the diversity in organizational strategies and actions that we observed. The participating L&D units were implementing QI processes with the goal of achieving strong and sustainable team-based care in their care-delivery processes. Such diversity in implementation approaches is consistent with the QI model, which recognizes that any given organization must craft an implementation strategy that works best for the unique circumstances within which it operates. Even with such diversity, however, all the participating L&D units were striving to achieve adoption of the set of competencies and practices defined in the MedTeams and TeamSTEPPS models.

We summarized our findings regarding each of the research questions at the end of Chapter Three (for the process evaluation) and Chapter Four (for the outcome evaluation), so these findings are not repeated here. Rather, we synthesize the combined sets of findings, to examine the relationships between the L&D units' implementation processes and associated outcomes. In Table 5.1, we delineate the key implementation methods used by each L&D unit, characterize each unit's progress in adopting teamwork practices, and list the effects on outcomes observed for that unit. It is in this synthesis that we address the two study objectives together—(1) to understand what is required for L&D units to achieve sustainable teamwork practices that (2) can influence outcomes of the care provided by the units. We group the five sites according to whether they had pursued teamwork improvements before this study began, to allow ready comparisons between the two groups.

These results allow us to draw some conclusions from what we have learned and to explore areas in which further work may be needed to expand our understanding of these processes. The experiences of these L&D units indicate that it is possible, by pursuing a proactive strategy, to make substantial progress in one year of implementing teamwork practices, and to affect proximal outcomes, such as staff knowledge and perceptions. This is shown in particular

Table 5.1
Summary of Results Regarding Implementation Progress and Outcome Changes, by Site

Result	No Previous Work on Teamwork			Previously Worked on Teamwork	
	Site 1	Site 3	Site 5	Site 2	Site 4
Baseline status	No work	No work	No work	Work	Work
Implementation actions					
Proactive strategy[a]	xxx	x	xx	xx	x
Active implementation team[a]	xxx	xx	xx	xx	x
Had a facilitator	x			x	
Trained all staff	x			x	
Used ongoing coaching	x	x		x	
Practices implemented[b]	8	3	3	4	3
Observed teamwork practices[c]	3.3–4.0	2.8–3.0	3.4–3.9	3.7–4.1	4.5–4.6
Outcome changes					
Staff perceptions improved	5	1	4	3	3
Reduction in AOI				x	

[a] x = weak. xx = moderate. xxx = strong.

[b] Of a total of nine teamwork practices.

[c] Observed at the end of the study; average scores out of a total of five points.

by the results for site 1, which used a very proactive and structured strategy that included all the actions identified in this study as important to effect change. Even with a less proactive approach, the other two sites that had not previously pursued teamwork improvements (site 3 and site 5) made progress, but they implemented fewer teamwork practices, used fewer implementation techniques, and had weaker improvements in staff perceptions. However, we did not find reductions in adverse events for patients for any of these three sites.

We found quite different results for the two sites that already had carried out teamwork improvements before the study. Site 2 pursued a moderately proactive strategy, including use of the key implementation actions, whereas site 4 had a more passive, incremental approach. Yet, the observation study gave both sites high scores for their teamwork practices. At the same time, both sites had some improvements in staff teamwork knowledge and perceptions, and site 2 showed a decline in adverse outcomes for patients.

Looking across all five sites, it becomes apparent that more than one year of implementation effort is required to achieve a high level of performance on teamwork practices. All of the sites reported at the end of the study that their work was not yet done and that they intended to continue their work on teamwork improvements. The scores the five sites received in the observation study support this premise. The two sites that already had worked on teamwork prior to the study had higher observation scores than any of the three sites that started work during the study year, which also supports the conclusion that more than one year is needed to reach that level of performance.

These combined results suggest that two dynamics might be involved in the second (or later) years of teamwork implementation. First, momentum gained from the first year of implementation might continue into later years, such that subsequent, more-limited implementation actions might reinforce that momentum toward continued improvement. This premise is supported by the high scores that sites 2 and 4 had in the observation study. Second, it might not be possible to sustain a high level of intensity in implementation beyond the first year of work. Thus, the strategies of these two sites might reasonably represent what could be expected of levels of activity for later years.

Implications

The study results reinforce the importance of developing and implementing a well-crafted strategy, which includes training staff in the L&D units, working with staff to introduce practices, and providing coaching on the effective use of those practices. We see this result in Table 5.1. We also heard these messages in the retrospective assessments by the participating L&D units, including the importance of persevering in the pursuit of their strategy over time (summarized in Chapter Three).

These findings are consistent with the guidance provided by AHRQ on its TeamSTEPPS website (AHRQ, undated). AHRQ emphasizes several organizational factors that are required for success. Perhaps the most important of these is readiness to change—genuine commitment from the hospital and department leadership. Others include a committed physician champion in the unit, an interdisciplinary implementation team to encourage buy-in and lead actions, a physical environment that is conducive to team interactions, and regular self-assessments of progress. These factors are not unique; they have consistently been found to be essential for successful quality improvement of any type.

The limited effects on patient outcomes are one of the disappointing results from the study, given that we analyzed outcomes using trend data over seven or more three-month quarters. Although small numbers of events could be a reason for the negative results, we used the AOI to manage this issue by aggregating ten types of adverse events. We chose to use the AOI because it could be measured using administrative data. Future work could benefit by exploring possible effects on other clinical measures. The successes reported by the participating L&D units during the study suggested that their work was having effects on their care delivery for patients, which pointed to possible candidates for other measures. For example, outcomes the sites cited as being affected by their teamwork-improvement efforts included emergency C-sections, C-section infection rates, and customer-satisfaction scores.

We did find improvements on the perceptions and knowledge of L&D unit staff regarding teamwork practices, and we identified key implementation actions that appeared to influence those improvements. Staff experiences represent an important outcome measure, which would be useful not only for research but also for L&D units implementing teamwork improvement, to help them assess their progress. In Chapter Two, we noted the relatively low response rates we obtained for the staff surveys as a limitation of the study. However, the changes we found were in the expected direction, which gives us confidence in these results.

This study has identified a set of key factors that need to be included in a given strategy for teamwork improvement, in particular, provision of teamwork training for all staff, ongoing coaching, and use of a facilitator to support implementation. However, the results do not point to a standard template for an implementation strategy that other L&D units could pursue with little adaptation to their unique circumstances. This result is consistent with the principles of quality improvement. The implication is that there may not be one fixed "intervention" that could be tested in comparative-control studies to develop further evidence for teamwork practices.

As described in Chapter Two, we selected L&D units for the study that had made a commitment to achieving teamwork improvement, with the rationale that successful adoption of new practices takes work and perseverance and those who are not strongly committed are not likely to make progress because they lack the perseverance to continue working the implementation process. This premise was supported by the insights obtained from the participating L&D units, which highlighted the need for such commitment to make progress. Therefore, the reference group we identify for generalizability is other L&D units that also are committed to making such improvements.

In assessing the validity and generalizability of the results of the study, we draw on the work of Silverman and associates (1990), which distinguishes between internal and external validity. When considered in qualitative research, the term *validity* refers to the "best available approximation of the truth or falsity of propositions, including propositions about cause." *Internal validity* refers to the degree of confidence one has that a posited relationship between two or more factors is true—that the factors are causally related. *External validity* refers to the extent to which the findings of research can be generalized to other persons, places, times, or settings beyond the entities involved in a study (Silverman, Ricci, and Gunter, 1990).

We have confidence in the internal validity of the results of this study and the conclusions we have drawn from them. This confidence is based on the rich information obtained on the dynamics of implementation processes, our identification of common themes that run across the diverse approaches taken by the five participating L&D units, and our ability to triangulate findings across the various types of data we collected. We recognize, however, that there may be some uncertainty regarding the external validity of the results—that is, the extent to which these case-study results can be generalized to a larger population of L&D units.

It is possible that, if other L&D units were observed as additional case studies, some different factors or strategies might emerge that also influence implementation success. We encourage further work in this area to test these findings with additional case studies, which could help build a depth of evidence across a larger number of organizations.

Tools and Strategies for Teamwork

The material in this appendix is drawn from the DoD TeamSTEPPS program.

Tools

Team Huddle

The team huddle is a tool for reinforcing the plans already in place for treating patients and for assessing the need to change plans. It serves as a tool for developing a shared understanding between team members of the plan of care. It also provides team leaders with an opportunity to informally monitor patient- and unit-level situations.

Team huddles are

- brief
- informal
- information-sharing sessions between team members.

Team huddles require team members to

- meet at predetermined or ad hoc intervals
- assess all pertinent information
- summarize actions to be taken
- revise action plans as needed.

Anyone can request a team huddle.

It is important to point out that team leaders and team members can use information gathered during team huddles for resource management. Given specific situations that may arise, team leaders may choose to reallocate resources or redelegate team members to specific situational needs.

Team huddles provide core-team members with an opportunity to discuss changes in patients' conditions and potential changes to plans of care. For example, changes in a patient's condition can be discussed during a brief team huddle called by a nurse. Team members can then discuss potential revisions to patient care that may result from the changes in the patient's condition. Team huddles are also important in the sharing of departmental information. For instance, a nurse who is treating a patient with a severely infected wound to the knee might become aware of delay in the blood labs resulting from centrifuge maintenance. This nurse would share this departmental information with his or her fellow core-team members. The group can then decide whether the patient's plan of care should be altered.

Debriefs

Debriefs serve as a tool for promoting teamwork and enhancing team performance. Debriefs can be used to ensure that information seeking, information sharing, and monitoring are taking place among team members and that team members are assessing their performance and to develop learning based on teamwork skills and not a clinical case.

Debriefs help team members assess their performance as a team both after a crisis and at the end of the day. Debriefs are a developmental tool that serve a dual purpose in that they help identify good work and mistakes in the care of a patient. Debriefs help reinforce good performance using real-life, recent situations and case studies. Debriefs also allow for collective learning because they require team-member participation. As a developmental tool, they do not require much time. Debriefs should be conducted to help develop team skills and identify breakdowns in teamwork that have had an impact on patient care.

Anyone on the team can request a debrief.

Debriefs should be conducted for the following reasons:

- so team members learn from actual situations
- so learning takes place collectively
- so team members can exchange information
- so teams can improve performance.

STEP

How do we "monitor the situation"? What components of the situation provide relevant cues? A STEP assessment involves ongoing/continual assessment of the following:

- the status of the patient
- the team members
- the environment
- the progress toward the goal.

Status of the Patient. Perhaps the most obvious component of the situation that requires monitoring and continual assessment in the health-care setting is the status of the patient.

The patient is the central focus of the medical situation. The condition of the patient may dynamically change. Small changes in the patient's vital signs may dramatically alter the tasks that the team needs to perform, as well as the urgency with which they must be performed.

To assess the status of the patient, consider the following:

- patient history (e.g., previous illnesses, family's medical history)
- vital signs (e.g., blood pressure)
- medications
- physical exam
- plan of care
- psychological condition (e.g., stress level of the patient).

Team Members. *Team members* refers to paying attention to one's team members—e.g., their needs, stress level, workload, and future tasks.

Recognizing that everyone is fallible and that health-care providers are just as prone to human error as the general population, teams that maintain an awareness of their individual members' functioning are more likely to catch mistakes or oversights shortly after they occur and are, therefore, more likely to "fix" the situation before it escalates and causes harm to the patient.

To assess the team, consider the following for each team member:

- fatigue (this includes physical fatigue, as well as vigilance fatigue)
- workload (workload can affect an individual team member's functioning and stress level, for example)
- task performance
- skill level
- stress level.

This is not about conducting a performance appraisal or "spying" on co-workers and teammates. It is about providing a safety net to the team and ensuring that any mistakes or oversights are caught quickly and can be rectified easily before they become major issues. It is about "watching each other's back."

In the medical environment, training and work involve long hours, sleep deprivation, situations of extreme stress, and irregular eating habits. However, safe patient care mandates that providers ensure that they are all fit and ready to fulfill their duties. Besides monitoring one's team members, it is also important to monitor oneself and make sure that one is also fit and ready to fulfill your duties. "I'M SAFE" is a simple checklist that should be used daily (or more frequently) to determine each team member's readiness to perform, especially if quality and patient safety could be compromised:

- illness: Am I feeling so bad that I do not have or cannot maintain that critical edge I need to perform my duties?
- medication: Is any medication I am taking while working affecting my ability to maintain that critical edge?
- stress: Is there something (a life event or situation at work) affecting me so I cannot focus on performing my duties or affecting my ability to maintain that critical edge?
- alcohol/drugs: Is the use of alcohol or illicit drugs affecting me so I cannot focus on performing my duties or affecting my ability to maintain that critical edge?
- fatigue: Am I getting enough sleep so that I can focus on performing my duties and maintain my critical edge?
- eating, elimination, and emotions
  - eating: Many times, we are so focused on ensuring that our patients' basic human needs are met that we forget about taking care of our own. This category addresses that fact. Each of us must maintain an appropriate blood-sugar level to think and perform.
  - elimination: You may not realize it, but not seeing to our elimination needs affects our ability to concentrate and stresses us physiologically.
  - emotions: Am I upset or angry about something that has happened in either my personal or work life?

Environment. *Environment* refers to all the environmental conditions or elements that can affect the team's attainment of the goal. The environment consists of more than the immediate context of the one doctor/one nurse/one technician/one patient situation; it also consists of the environment of the unit as a whole. An individual patient's plan of care may be affected by what is happening in the greater context of the unit (e.g., an influx of patients onto the unit). The environment may directly affect the approaches or timing of specific care to maximize the needs of all the teams and patients.

To assess the environment, consider the following:

- facility information (e.g., number of operating rooms, number of beds on the unit)
- administrative information (e.g., number of patients recently admitted)
- human resources (e.g., number and qualifications of staff on the floor)
- triage acuity
- equipment (e.g., proper functioning of equipment).

Progress Toward the Goal. *Progress toward the goal* refers to where the team is with respect to its goal. With respect to health care, the team's goal is to ensure the patient's health and well-being.

In dynamic, fast-paced environments (such as those that medical teams face), frequently monitoring and assessing the team's progress toward the goal will enable the team to identify, in real time, when performance gaps emerge or when the team moves in the wrong direction. In turn, the team can self-correct and select a more appropriate course or plan of care for the patient.

To assess progress, consider the following:

- What is the status of the team's patients?
- What is the goal of the team?
- What tasks/actions have been completed or need to be done?
- Is the plan still appropriate?

Two-Challenge Rule

A specific strategy for providing spoken support, addressing conflict, and preventing errors is the two-challenge rule. This tool was originally developed by human-factors experts to help airline captains prevent disasters caused by momentary lapses of judgment by otherwise-excellent decisionmakers.

In addition to requesting clarification and confirmation from team members when potentially ambiguous situations arise, each team member should also challenge a colleague if he or she feels that any action may jeopardize patient safety. It is important to voice one's concern at least twice, since the initial assertion may be ignored.

If the issue is not resolved after the two challenges, a stronger course of action should be taken (e.g., the organization's conflict-resolution policy, chain of command).

The two-challenge rule will be most effective if team members do the following:

- Provide the first challenge in the form of a respectful question.
- Provide information to support the concern in the second challenge.

If concerns are raised (one is challenged), the person challenged has the responsibility to acknowledge the concerns and not ignore them.

Feedback

Feedback is one form of spoken mutual support. Feedback can be

- formal or informal (e.g., provided during a scheduled meeting or casually during a team huddle)
- provided by anyone on the team, regardless of rank.

Types of Feedback. *Constructive* feedback is considerate and task-specific and focuses attention on the performance and not on the individual. *Evaluative* feedback helps the individual understand the performance information by comparing behavior to standards or to the individual's own past performance. Do not compare the individual's performance to that of other team members; instead, if possible, use past performance as a guide for the feedback.

When to Use Constructive and Evaluative Feedback. Constructive feedback is often provided by *all team members* regardless of their role on the team. It is most beneficial when it is focused on team processes and is provided regularly. Evaluative feedback, on the other hand, is most often provided by individuals in a mentoring or coaching role. The coach may compare the individual's performance to that person's past performance to demonstrate how much the individual has improved. In addition, evaluative feedback may be used to compare the individual's performance with established standards, as in the case of preparing for licensure or certifications.

When providing feedback to others, it is important to make certain that feedback is delivered in a *timely* fashion, is *directed toward behaviors*, is *specific*, provides *direction for improvement*, and is *considerate*.

- Make sure to provide feedback in a timely fashion. Feedback that is not timely will have less impact on performance. Feedback is most effective if the receiver can easily associate the executed behavior with the feedback.
- Make sure that feedback is provided in behavioral terms and not in personal terms. Never attribute a team member's poor performance to internal factors. Such destructive feedback lowers self-efficacy and subsequent performance.
- If applicable, make sure to specify what behaviors need correcting. Imagine that you are receiving feedback from a peer who tells you that your surgical techniques need work. Such a statement is too general to enable the listener to improve. The person receiving feedback will be better able to correct or modify performance if specific actions are mentioned during feedback.
- If applicable, provide directions for improvement.
- Remember to consider team members' feelings when delivering feedback. When delivering feedback, remember to praise good performance. The message will seem less critical if information is supplied about what the person did well along with information on how he or she can improve. Fairness and respect will also cushion the effect of any negative feedback.
- Feedback can also be provided to reinforce good performance. Everyone benefits from knowing that they have done a good job and that others have recognized it.

Strategies

DESC Script (Describe, Express, Suggest, Consequences)

What if the conflict has become personal in nature? The DESC script may be used to manage all types of conflict; however, it may be especially useful in resolving affective conflict.

- Describe the specific situation or behavior, providing concrete data.
- Express how the situation makes you feel.
- Suggest other alternatives and seek agreement.
- Consequences should be stated in terms of impact on performance goals. Individuals should strive for consensus.

SBAR (Situation, Background, Assessment, Recommendation)

SBAR is a strategy that team members may use to communicate clearly and concisely. The abbreviation illustrates the type of information that should be communicated to physicians and other providers.

Check-Backs

The check-back strategy addresses closed-loop communication, which is a specific aspect of information exchange. Closed-loop communication ensures that the receiver understands the information as intended.

The check-back strategy requires a verification of information. This strategy is used frequently in aviation (known as "read-back") as aviators verify critical information, such as headings and altitudes.

The steps include the sender initiating the message, the receiver accepting it and providing feedback, and the sender double-checking or verifying that the message was received as intended.

The Joint Commission requires the use of check-backs. It requires that anyone taking a telephone or spoken order or diagnostic test that the organization determines to be "critical" write it down and read it back ("write it down and read it back" requirement).

Hand-Offs

When a team member steps out or leaves at the end of a shift, there is a risk that necessary information about the patient might not be communicated. There is also a slight lapse in coverage when someone goes on a break or goes to check on another patient and does not communicate his or her whereabouts or provide any updates on the patients.

The hand-off strategy is designed to enhance information exchange at critical times, such as shift changes and breaks. It consists of the following steps:

- Notify team members when stepping out for a moment or ending a shift, and update the whiteboard.
- Convey all necessary information about the patient and his or her status to the medical professionals taking over the next shift.
- Update the whiteboard with patient's status.
- Communicate information to secretary and charge nurse.
- Alert the team that a hand-off has occurred.

When handing off care to another team member, be sure to close the communication loop by verifying that the teammate is accepting the hand-off. Using this strategy can help build a shared mental model for the individuals taking over the shift (i.e., they know the information about the patients and the plans of care). A hand-off should occur during transitions of patient care. Examples include the following:

- shift change
- break times
- transfer of the patient to another setting, department, or provider.

It is important to note that, when a patient is transferred, a complete list of medications must be provided to the new provider. This requirement is part of the Joint Commission's medication-reconciliation patient-safety goal (see Joint Commission, 2010, for more details).

To complete a successful hand-off, the team member should communicate the following information:

- patient's history, status, and plan of care (e.g., critical and scheduled for surgery)
- provider coverage (e.g., Dr. Smith will be doing the surgery)
- workload level (e.g., how many patients there are and who is covering them)
- provider availability (e.g., how many physicians and other medical professionals are available)
- facility information (e.g., equipment and other material resources).

Call-Outs

Calling out is a technique used to provide information to all team members in an efficient manner. Important or critical information is announced to the whole team during emergencies and at other times when information must be passed in a timely manner.

The team members can then anticipate their next steps and are able to adapt more quickly to a rapidly changing situation. The use of call-outs can also assist the team member who is recording the events during an emergency.

Matrix of Questions and Stakeholders for Site Visits

Table B.1 contains the questions and stakeholders for our site visits.

Table B.1
Longitudinal Labor and Delivery Teamwork Study

Question	Implementation Team	Physicians, Any Specialty	Nursing Staff	Clerical Staff	Individual Leaders	NICU Staff
1. Hospital environment for quality and safety						
1.1. To what extent does your *hospital* have a patient-safety culture?	X	X	X	X	X	X
1.2. Does your hospital have patient-safety standards that are documented in protocols or guidelines? If yes, please describe them.	X	X	X	X	X	X
1.3. Does the hospital support efforts that improve patient safety? How?	X	X	X	X	X	X
1.4–1.6. What type of reporting system for errors or adverse events does the hospital have? *[If has a system]* What types of events are reported in the system? *[If has a system]* How would you rate the overall effectiveness of the event- or error-reporting system in improving patient safety in your organization?	X					
1.7. To what extent has the hospital placed an emphasis on meeting quality performance standards? developed effective structure and process to support quality improvement? involved staff in making changes for quality improvement? implemeneted a management style that supports quality improvement?	X					
2. Patient-safety culture in the L&D unit						
2.1. How does your *L&D unit* differ from the hospital in patient-safety culture?	X	X	X		X	X

Table B.1—Continued

Question	Implementation Team	Physicians, Any Specialty	Nursing Staff	Clerical Staff	Individual Leaders	NICU Staff
2.2. A set of 8 steps of change has been identified as required to create a patient-safety culture. Where is your *L&D unit* in each of these steps? 　Create sense of urgency 　Build the guiding team 　Develop change vision and strategy 　Gain understanding and buy-in 　Empower others 　Achieve short-term wins 　Don't let up; be relentless 　Create a new culture	x					
2.3. What strategy and actions are being taken in your L&D unit to create a stronger patient-safety culture?	x	x	x	x		x
2.4. Does your *L&D unit* have patient-safety standards that are documented in protocols or guidelines? If yes, please describe them. 　a. How are these protocols or guidelines disseminated within the unit? 　b. Are the protocols or guidelines clear and easy for all staff to understand?	x	x	x	x		x
2.5. What factors are facilitating the progress you have made in creating a stronger patient-safety culture in the L&D unit?	x	x	x	x	x	x
2.6. What factors are slowing your progress in strengthening patient-safety culture?	x	x	x	x	x	x
3. Hospital leadership support for L&D teamwork						
3.1. To what extent has the *leadership of the hospital* been involved in each of the following aspects of your L&D teamwork activities? 　Shaping the project vision 　Planning for start-up 　Making revisions or changes during implementation 　Requesting project updates from the project team 　Providing guidance and feedback to the project team 　Assisting in removing barriers to implementation 　Promoting/marketing the project	x				x	

Table B.1—Continued

Question	Implementation Team	Physicians, Any Specialty	Nursing Staff	Clerical Staff	Individual Leaders	NICU Staff
3.2. Has the **hospital leadership** provided the project team with adequate time to carry out tasks related to the project? adequate funding to carry out the project? autonomy to carry out the project?	x				x	
4. The teamwork-improvement team						
4.1. How many and what types of staff are serving as trainers and coaches as teamwork improvements have been implemented in your L&D unit? What is the ratio of trainers to unit staff for physicians, nurses, and other staff?	x					
4.2. Which of the following are represented **on the teamwork implementation team?**	x					
4.3. How does the implementation team operate in terms of frequency and content of meetings roles and responsibilities of each member approach to decisionmaking communications among team members between meetings	x				x	
4.4. Has the team prepared an implementation plan for L&D teamwork improvement? a. When was the plan first prepared? b. Was it reviewed by staff before finalizing it? c. Has the plan been finalized? d. Has it been revised or updated since then? If so, when?	x				x	
4.5. Does the implementation plan include the following? A statement of goals and overall strategy Specification of actions designed to achieve the goals Designation of the staff who have lead and support responsibilities for each action A timetable for completion of each action Process measures to assess the extent to which actions were in fact implemented successfully as planned	x					
4.6. How does the implementation team work with the plan as the teamwork implementation activities move forward?	x					

Table B.1—Continued

Question	Implementation Team	Physicians, Any Specialty	Nursing Staff	Clerical Staff	Individual Leaders	NICU Staff
4.7. What actions has the implementation team taken to build a sense of teamwork among multidisciplinary team members? What has been the team's experience in achieving teamwork and cross-disciplinary respect and participation?	x				x	
4.8. As challenges have arisen during implementation, how has the team responded to the challenges to ensure continued progress toward the teamwork goals?	x				x	
4.9. To what extent has the implementation team felt empowered by the L&D unit's leadership to make change? What about the hospital's leadership?	x				x	
5. Teamwork training for the L&D unit staff						
5.1. How have the local trainers/coaches been trained to provide effective teamwork-improvement support to the L&D unit staff? Length of training; Date(s) when the training was conducted; Training content; Role-playing to learn techniques; Timing of training relative to start of teamwork improvement in the unit	x					
5.2. What additional training, skills, or information would the trainers/coaches feel they need to enable them to function effectively in training and coaching unit staff on teamwork?	x				x	
5.3. How is (or was) the initial training for the L&D unit staff conducted? Date(s) when the training was conducted; Length of each training session; Number of training sessions; Who did the training at the sessions; What content was covered in the sessions; Percentage of unit staff who received the training	x	x	x	x		x

Table B.1—Continued

Question	Implementation Team	Physicians, Any Specialty	Nursing Staff	Clerical Staff	Individual Leaders	NICU Staff
5.4. Have follow-up training sessions been conducted, or are any planned for the future? What is the purpose of the follow-up sessions? To train those who did not attend the first sessions, to refresh earlier training? When were the training sessions conducted, or when are they planned?	x				x	
5.5. Were the staff asked to complete evaluations of the training? If so, what were their assessments of the usefulness and value of the training?	x	x	x	x		x
5.6. Was staff knowledge of teamwork tested before and after the training to assess training's effect on teamwork knowledge? If so, what effects were found?	x					
6. Implementing teamwork improvements						
Overall implementation status						
6.1. How is your teamwork implementation progressing relative to what was specified in the implementation plan?	x				x	
6.2. To what extent have you changed the L&D team structure as part of teamwork improvements? a. What changes were made, and why were they made? b. How well is the new structure working?	x				x	
6.3. Which aspects of the teamwork model have been implemented in your L&D unit, and what were your experiences in implementing them? Leadership Situation monitoring Mutual support Communication	x	x	x		x	x
6.4. Overall, please rate the current status regarding how well each aspect of teamwork has been implemented in your L&D unit.	x	x	x	x	x	x

Table B.1—Continued

Question	Implementation Team	Physicians, Any Specialty	Nursing Staff	Clerical Staff	Individual Leaders	NICU Staff
6.5–6.14. Are you using each of the following as a teamwork tool? The team huddle Debriefs STEP Feedback The two-challenge rule DESC script Collaboration SBAR Call-outs Check-backs	x	x	x	x		x
6.15. Are you using hand-off techniques?	x	x	x	x		x
6.16. For each teamwork tool, please identify whether the tool has been integrated into routine practice, and rate how well your L&D unit is using the tool when it is used.	x					
6.17. Have your coaches completed a coaching self-assessment addressing the 13 competencies that are important for fulfilling the coaching role successfully? a. If yes, have self-assessments been done more than once? Has there been improvement in coaching skills? b. If no, would the coaches complete the TMA self-assessment at each site visit?	x					
6.18. What issues or challenges have most affected coaches' ability to fulfill their coaching responsibilities? How have these issues been managed?	x				x	
6.19. What are the greatest successes achieved through the coaching? What factors contributed to those successes?	x				x	

Table B.1—Continued

Question	Implementation Team	Physicians, Any Specialty	Nursing Staff	Clerical Staff	Individual Leaders	NICU Staff
Assessment of L&D teamwork performance						

6.20. How well are staff performing as team members on the following dimensions?
  Clear understanding of role
  Clearly defined responsibilities
  High level of commitment
  Good understanding of culture, norms
  Shared mental models
  Effective use of teamwork behaviors
  Communication of patient information
  Attitudes needed for team mutual trust
  Respond to feedback with change
  Work with coach to improve
  Well-aligned expectations for team
  Adaptive and reactive team
  High motivation and morale
	x	x	x	x	x	x

6.21. What issues have you faced that have been important barriers to achieving effective teamwork in your L&D unit? How have you worked to manage these barriers?
  Inconsistent team membership
  Lack of time
  Lack of information sharing
  Hierarchy
  Defensiveness
  Conventional thinking
  Varying communication styles
  Conflict
  Lack of coordination and follow-up with co-workers
  Distractions
  Fatigue
  Workload
  Misinterpretation of cues
  Lack of role clarity
	x	x	x	x	x	x

6.22. What have been your greatest successes thus far in achieving effective teamwork in your L&D unit?	x	x	x	x	x	x

Table B.1—Continued

Question	Implementation Team	Physicians, Any Specialty	Nursing Staff	Clerical Staff	Individual Leaders	NICU Staff
7. Concluding questions						
7.1. In what ways is the larger hospital environment affecting your progress in achieving stronger teamwork in the L&D unit, either positively or negatively? What are the implications for your ability to achieve teamwork improvement?	×	×	×		×	×
7.2. How is the external environment affecting the L&D teamwork activities, either directly on the L&D unit or indirectly through effects on the overall hospital? What are the implications for your ability to achieve teamwork improvement?	×	×	×		×	×
7.3. How does your actual experience in teamwork improvement compare to what you expected as you started the initiative? What are the biggest surprises?	×				×	
7.4. What advice would you give to other L&D units to enhance their success in improving teamwork?	×	×	×	×	×	×

Monthly Update Teleconference: Longitudinal Labor and Delivery Teamwork Study

MONTHLY UPDATE TELECONFERENCE
Longitudinal Labor and Delivery Teamwork Study

Hospital: _____   RAND Staff: _____

Date of call: _____

1.   Please give us a brief overview of the highlights of your teamwork enhancement activities during the past month (for the first update, up until this date).

THE TEAMWORK IMPROVEMENT TEAM

2.   What are the current roles and status of your trainers and coaches for teamwork improvement?

3.   Which of the following are represented *on the teamwork implementation team*? (Check all that apply)

☐ Senior hospital management
☐ Senior medical management of the labor and delivery unit
☐ Staff designated as trainers
☐ Other OB/gynecology physicians
☐ Other anesthesiologists
☐ Other neonatologists
☐ Other nurses, nurse practitioners, or physician's assistants
☐ Patients
☐ Community stakeholders
☐ Others (specify)

4.   Have you changed the L&D team structure since it was first organized? If so, how?

5.   Has the team prepared an implementation plan for L&D teamwork improvement? How did you approach development of the plan? How has the plan been modified, if at all, since you first prepared it?

TEAMWORK TRAINING FOR THE L&D UNIT STAFF

6.   What is the status of the initial training for the L&D unit staff?

7.   Have follow-up training sessions been conducted or are any planned for the future? What is the purpose of the follow-up sessions?

ORGANIZATIONAL CONTEXT: PATIENT SAFETY CULTURE AND TEAMWORK

8.   What strategy and actions are being taken in your labor and delivery unit to create a stronger patient safety culture?

9.   To what extent has the *leadership of the hospital* been involved in your L&D unit's activities to strengthen teamwork in the delivery process?

IMPLEMENTING TEAMWORK IMPROVEMENTS

10.   How is your teamwork implementation progressing relative to what was specified in the implementation plan?

11.   What is your status in implementing each of the four components of the teamwork model in your L&D unit? What have been your experiences in implementing them?

Teamwork Component	Current Status and Experiences
Leadership: including effective leaders, resource management, team huddle, debriefs, conflict resolution, effective teamwork	
Situation monitoring: including situation awareness, shared mental model, cross monitoring, patient monitoring, team member monitoring, environment monitoring, progress toward goal	
Mutual support: including task assistance, good feedback, two-challenge rule, DESC script, collaboration for conflict resolution	
Communications: including SBAR, call-out, check-back, handoff	

12. Which of the teamwork tools are you working with, or plan to use, as listed below:

Teamwork Tool	Already Done	Working on It	Plan to Use	Don't Know
Team huddle				
Debriefs				
STEP				
Feedback				
The two-challenge rule				
DESC script				
Collaboration				
SBAR				
Call-outs				
Check-backs				
Handoff techniques				

13. What is the status of coaching activities by your trainers, as they are working with the unit staff?

SUCCESSES AND CHALLENGES

14. What have been your greatest successes and challenges in the most recent period of implementing teamwork in the L&D unit?

Greatest Successes	What Helped to Succeed

Greatest Challenges	Responses to the Challenges

Questions for Final Assessment: Longitudinal Labor and Delivery Teamwork Study

QUESTIONS FOR FINAL ASSESSMENT
Longitudinal Labor and Delivery Teamwork Study

Hospital: _____   Date: _____

Lead Team Members Participating: _____

_____

ENVIRONMENTAL EFFECTS ON TEAMWORK IMPLEMENTATION

1. **How much did each of the following environmental factors affect your progress in implementing improved teamwork practices?**

    Overall hospital's patient safety culture and support for patient safety actions

    Patient safety culture and support for patient safety actions in the L&D unit

    Other quality or performance initiatives introduced by the hospital or L&D unit

    Changes in the hospital's operating or computer systems

    Renovations or other changes to the hospital building that affected the L&D unit

    Changes in the leadership of the hospital or L&D unit

    Physical configuration of the L&D unit

    Other factors?

EFFECTS OF PROCESS FACTORS ON TEAMWORK IMPLEMENTATION

2. **How much did each of the following process factors affect your progress in implementing improved teamwork practices?**

    Support for teamwork improvement by the leadership of the hospital

    Involvement of leadership of the hospital in the implementation

    Receptivity of physicians, nurses, and other L&D unit staff

    Communications technology (e.g., telephones, beepers)

    Staff turnover in the L&D unit

    Size and fluctuations in L&D patient volume and related workload

    Other factors?

THE TEAMWORK IMPLEMENTATION TEAM

3. **How would you advise other L&D units (or any other type of unit) regarding the importance, role, and activities of an implementation team that guides the teamwork improvement work?**

    Team size and types of professional disciplines that should be on it

    The most important functions the team should be performing

    How frequently the team should meet

    Methods used for decision making and consensus building within the team

    How the team gets input and feedback from staff on the unit during implementation

    Planning the content and schedule of the implementation work

    Communications among team members between meetings

    Other items?

4. **How important was it to have a physician leader or champion for the work?**

5. **How important was it to have a person designated to facilitate the work of the implementation team and the conduct of the teamwork improvement activities?**

6. **As challenges arose during teamwork implementation, how did the team respond to them to ensure continued progress toward the teamwork goals?**

TEAMWORK TRAINING AND COACHING

7. **Based on your experiences, what are the best approaches for conducting initial training of the L&D unit staff on the teamwork model and practices?**

8. **What have you found to be the best ways to provide ongoing guidance and feedback to unit staff as they learn to work within the teamwork model and to use the individual teamwork practices involved?**

    Roles of formally designated coaches

    Other designated staff positions equivalent to a coach

    Reinforcement by unit leaders for physicians, nurses, others

    Periodic involvement of outside consultants to provide expert feedback

    Other methods?

9. **Based on your experiences thus far, what have been the most effective approaches for conducting refresher teamwork training?**

    For existing employees or physician staff

    For new employees or physician staff

IMPLEMENTING TEAMWORK IMPROVEMENTS

10. **The teamwork model encompasses the four components listed below. Based on your implementation experiences, how would you advise other organizations regarding which of these components to work on first and how to approach each of them. Which of the components have you found to be the most important to address?**

    Leadership

    Situation monitoring

    Mutual support

    Communications

11. **The teamwork model also provides guidance on use of the specific practices listed below. Again, based on your experiences, how would you advise other organizations regarding which of them to introduce first and how to approach working with them?**

    Is it necessary to adopt all of these practices?

    Which have been the most important practices for your L&D unit?

    How can team rounds about all patients and huddles about one patient be used most effectively?

Team huddle (team rounds)	Collaboration
Debrief	SBAR
Situation awareness	Call-out
Feedback	Check-back
Two-challenge rule	Handoff
DESC script	

12. **How have you approached engaging each of the key clinical groups working on the L&D unit in adoption of teamwork practices, including physicians, residents, nurses, and others?**

13. **What would you identify to be the most important mechanisms (e.g., board rounds, designated physician leaders) you implemented to improve teamwork on the unit? Is(are) there one or more specific mechanisms that have anchored your approach to implementation?**

14. **What do you think would be the ideal physical environment to support effective teamwork practices (e.g., core team sections, nurses station location, etc.)**

15. **What have you learned about the importance of, and approaches to, continually reinforcing new teamwork practices over time? What has worked especially well for you? What has not worked?**

16. **How have your experiences in using teamwork practices differed when applying them in day-to-day care activities versus using them at more intense times of "crisis" that require fast actions for patient care?**

17. **If you could go back and start your implementation process all over again, how would you do it differently?**

CONCLUDING QUESTIONS

18. **Looking across your full implementation process thus far, what have been your greatest successes thus far in achieving effective teamwork in your L&D unit? What factors facilitated these successes?**

19. **What have been your greatest frustrations or disappointments relative to what you had hoped to achieve thus far? What contributed to these issues, and how would you advise others to avoid such problems?**

20. **How does your actual experience in teamwork improvement compare with what you expected as you started the initiative? What are the biggest surprises?**

21. **Taking into account everything we discussed here today, what overall advice would you give to other L&D units to enhance their success in improving teamwork?**

Team Performance Observation Tool

Team Performance Observation Tool

Hospital: _____

Date: _____ Time period: _____

Observer: _____

Unit census at start: _____

Rating Scale
(circle 1)
Please comment
if 1 or 2

1 = Very Poor
2 = Poor
3 = Acceptable
4 = Good
5 = Excellent

	Rating by Hour			
1. Team Structure	**Hour 1**	**Hour 2**	**Hour 3**	**Hour 4**
a. Assembles a team				
b. Establishes a leader				
c. Identifies team goals and vision				
d. Assigns roles and responsibilities				
e. Holds team members accountable				
f. Actively shares information among team members				
Comments:				
Overall Rating – Team Structure				
2. Leadership	**Rating**			
a. Utilizes resources efficiently to maximize team performance				
b. Balances workload within the team				
c. Delegates tasks or assignments, as appropriate				
d. Conducts briefs, huddles, and debriefs				
e. Empowers team members to speak freely and ask questions				
Comments:				
Overall Rating – Leadership				
3. Situation Monitoring	**Rating**			
a. Includes patient/family in communication				
b. Cross monitors fellow team members				
c. Applies the STEP process when monitoring the situation				
d. Fosters communication to ensure team members have a shared mental model				
Comments:				
Overall Rating – Situation Monitoring				
4. Mutual Support	**Rating**			
a. Provides task-related support				
b. Provides timely and constructive feedback to team members				
c. Effectively advocates for the patient				
d. Uses the Two-Challenge rule, CUS, and DESC script to resolve conflict				
e. Collaborates with team members				
Comments:				
Overall Rating – Mutual Support				
5. Communication	**Rating**			
a. Coaching feedback routinely provided to team members, when appropriate				
b. Provides brief, clear, specific and timely information to team members				
c. Seeks information from all available sources				
d. Verifies information that is communicated				
e. Uses SBAR, call-outs, check-backs and handoff techniques to communicate effectively with team members				
Comments:				
Overall Rating – Communication				
TEAM PERFORMANCE RATING				

Adapted from TeamSTEPPS 06.1   *Video Matrix*

Staff Survey Questionnaire

STAFF SURVEY
Labor and Delivery Teamwork

Thank you for taking part in this labor and delivery teamwork questionnaire. The purpose of the survey is to assess your views about the patient safety environment in the hospital and your labor and delivery unit, and to identify your perceptions and knowledge about teamwork in the labor and delivery unit.

Your participation is voluntary, and you do not have to answer any question you do not feel comfortable answering. If you prefer not to answer a specific question for any reason, you may leave it blank. You will not be evaluated on your answers to the questions. Answering the questions candidly will help improve future teamwork training.

RAND will use the survey results as part of a study to assess actions needed for a labor and delivery unit to achieve strong teamwork, and to examine how these actions relate to the perceptions of staff, improvements in practices, and patient outcomes. RAND will not have information that identifies you individually, and will combine your answers with data from other survey participants to report as aggregated statistics, totals, and averages.

Overall Hospital

Please circle a number from 1 to 5 to identify your agreement or disagreement with each question, using the following scale:

1 = strongly disagree; 2 = disagree; 3 = neither agree nor disagree; 4 = agree; 5 = strongly agree

Hospital management provides a work climate that promotes patient safety	1	2	3	4	5
The actions of hospital management show that patient safety is a top priority.	1	2	3	4	5
Hospital management seems interested in patient safety only after an adverse event happens.	1	2	3	4	5
Mistakes have led to positive changes here.	1	2	3	4	5
Things "fall between the cracks" when patients are transferred from one unit to another.	1	2	3	4	5
Problems often occur in the exchange of information across hospital units.	1	2	3	4	5
Hospital units work well together to provide the best care for patients.	1	2	3	4	5
We are actively doing things to improve patient safety.	1	2	3	4	5
After we make changes to improve patient safety, we evaluate their effectiveness.	1	2	3	4	5

The Labor and Delivery unit

Please circle a number from 1 to 5 to identify your agreement or disagreement with each question, using the following scale:

1 = strongly disagree; 2 = disagree; 3 = neither agree nor disagree; 4 = agree; 5 = strongly agree

The culture in this labor and delivery unit makes it easy to learn from the errors of others.	1	2	3	4	5
Medical errors are handled appropriately in this unit.	1	2	3	4	5
I know the proper channels to direct questions regarding patient safety in this unit.	1	2	3	4	5
I am encouraged by my colleagues to report any patient safety concerns I may have.	1	2	3	4	5
Staff feel like their mistakes are held against them.	1	2	3	4	5
When an event is reported, it feels like the person is being written up, not the problem.	1	2	3	4	5
Staff worry that mistakes they make are kept in their personnel file.	1	2	3	4	5
We have patient safety problems in this unit.	1	2	3	4	5
Patient safety is never sacrificed to get more work done.	1	2	3	4	5
Our procedures and systems are good at preventing errors from happening.	1	2	3	4	5
It is just by chance that more serious mistakes don't happen around here.	1	2	3	4	5

Patient safety grade

Please give your labor and delivery unit an overall grade on patient safety. Mark ONE answer.

O	O	O	O	O
A	B	C	D	E
Excellent	Very Good	Acceptable	Poor	Failing

Teamwork in Labor and Delivery

Please circle a number from 1 to 5 to identify your agreement or disagreement with each question, using the following scale:

1 = strongly disagree; 2 = disagree; 3 = neither agree nor disagree; 4 = agree; 5 = strongly agree

People support one another in this unit.	1	2	3	4	5
When a lot of work needs to be done quickly, we work together as a team to get the work done.	1	2	3	4	5
In this unit, people treat each other with respect.	1	2	3	4	5
When one area in this unit gets really busy, others help out..	1	2	3	4	5
The physicians and nurses here work together as a well-coordinated team.	1	2	3	4	5
Staff will freely speak up if they see something that may negatively affect patient care.	1	2	3	4	5
Staff feel free to question the decisions or actions of those with more authority.	1	2	3	4	5
Staff are afraid to ask questions when something does not seem right.	1	2	3	4	5
Disagreements in this unit are resolved appropriately (i.e., not *who* is right, but *what* is best for the patient)	1	2	3	4	5
I receive appropriate feedback about my performance.	1	2	3	4	5

Your Work Life

Please circle a number from 1 to 5 to identify your agreement or disagreement with each question, using the following scale:

1 = strongly disagree; 2 = disagree; 3 = neither agree nor disagree; 4 = agree; 5 = strongly agree

This hospital is a good place to work.	1	2	3	4	5
Morale in this unit is high.	1	2	3	4	5
Operating problems in the unit keep me from performing my best.	1	2	3	4	5
I feel like a respected member of the team in the unit.	1	2	3	4	5
I would rather not be working on this unit	1	2	3	4	5
My job is fulfilling professionally	1	2	3	4	5

Knowledge of Teamwork

Please answer the following questions by checking one box representing the **best** answer for each question.

1. What is the most frequently identified factor contributing to sentinel events (unexpected occurrence involving death or serious physical or psychological injury, or the risk thereof) in the United States?

☐ a. Inadequate documentation

☐ b. Inadequate communication

☐ c. Equipment malfunction or unavailability

☐ d. Inadequate training

☐ e. Unknown

2. Who on a team can initiate a team huddle?

☐ a. Team leader

☐ b. Physician

☐ c. Nurse

☐ d. Any team member

☐ e. Unknown

3. What are the characteristics of good feedback?

☐ a. Specific, firm, non-judgmental, and unplanned

☐ b. Friendly, non-judgmental, lenient, and supportive

☐ c. Timely, behavioral, specific, and non-judgmental

☐ d. Serious, authoritarian, correcting, and timely

☐ e. Unknown

4. What is situation awareness?

☐ a. Actively scanning behaviors and actions to assessment elements of the situation or environment

☐ b. Monitoring the actions of other team members for the purpose of sharing workload and reducing or avoiding errors

☐ c. Having a shared understanding of a situation or process among team members

☐ d. Having a state of knowing the current conditions affecting the team's work

☐ e. Unknown

5. Which of the following is (are) part of the role of a Team Leader?

☐ a. Make decisions through collective input of team members

☐ b. Empower team members to speak up and challenge

☐ c. Actively promote and facilitate good teamwork

☐ d. a and c only

☐ e. All of the above

☐ f. Unknown

6. What information exchange strategy informs all team members simultaneously during an emergency situation and helps team members anticipate next steps?

☐ a. SBAR

☐ b. Handoff

☐ c. Call-out

☐ d. Check-back

☐ e. Unknown

7. What is one of the most important reasons to share situation information with your team members?

☐ a. It provides a basis for predicting the behavior and needs of the team, and it facilitates decision making

☐ b. It fosters camaraderie among team members that facilitates social relationships outside the workplace

☐ c. It allows team members to determine how the team views their performance

☐ d. It provides team members with information needed to create work schedules

☐ e. Unknown

8. What is the primary purpose of a "debrief session" held after a particular case or event?

☐ a. To discuss strengths and weaknesses of the team and develop a plan for improvement

☐ b. To assess individual team members' performance

☐ c. To discuss individual team members' responsibilities

☐ d. To discuss the patient's status

☐ e. Unknown

About You

The following information will help in the analysis of the survey results.
Please mark ONE answer only for each question.

1. How long have you worked in this <u>hospital</u>?

    a. Less than 1 year   d. 11 to 15 years

    b. 1 to 5 years   e. 16 to 20 years

    c. 6 to 10 years   f. 21 years or more

2. How long have you worked in your current hospital <u>unit</u>?

    a. Less than 1 year   d. 11 to 15 years

    b. 1 to 5 years   e. 16 to 20 years

    c. 6 to 10 years   f. 21 years or more

3. What is your job status at the hospital?

    a. Full-time   c. Agency staff

    b. Part-time   d. contract staff

4. What is your staff position in this hospital? Mark ONE answer that best describes your staff position.

    a. Registered nurse   h. Pharmacist

    b. Physician assistant/nurse practitioner   i. Dietician

    c. LVN/LPN   j. Unit assistant/clerk/secretary

    d. Patient care assistant/aide/care partner   k. Therapist (e.g., respiratory, physical)

    e. OB/gynecology physician   l. Technician (e.g., EKG, lab, radiology)

    f. Anesthesiologist   m. Administration/management

    g. Resident physician, in training   n. Other, please specify:

5. How long have you worked in your current specialty or profession?

    a. Less than 1 year   d. 11 to 15 years

    b. 1 to 5 years   e. 16 to 20 years

    c. 6 to 10 years   f. 21 years or more

Regression Results for Staff Perceptions and Knowledge

Tables G.1–G.5 provide our regression results for staff perceptions and knowledge. In all five tables, SE indicates standard error. Each table shows the average positive response for items in a domain, where positive response is a response in either of the top two response categories. Site 3 is omitted as a reference site.

Table G.1
Regression Results for Staff Perceptions of Teamwork in the Labor and Delivery Unit

Result	Model 1			Model 2			Model 3			Model 4		
	Coefficient	Robust SE	p-Value	Coefficient	Robust SE	p-Value	Coefficient	Robust SE	p-Value	Coefficient	Robust SE	p-Value
Constant	0.627	0.012	<0.001	0.602	0.063	0.001	0.636	0.064	0.001	0.600	0.066	0.001
Wave 2	0.079	0.030	0.058	0.069	0.035	0.118				0.072	0.106	0.534
Site 1	0.173	0.006	<0.001	0.153	0.025	0.003	0.119	0.018	0.002	0.156	0.044	0.024
Site 2	0.036	0.004	0.001	0.025	0.017	0.212	-0.016	0.015	0.320	0.020	0.040	0.638
Site 4	0.230	0.005	<0.001	0.215	0.016	<0.001	0.182	0.008	<0.001	0.219	0.034	0.003
Site 5	-0.067	0.002	<0.001	-0.095	0.021	0.010	-0.191	0.020	0.001	-0.095	0.020	0.010
Time on unit 6–10 years				0.018	0.022	0.463	0.019	0.020	0.408	0.019	0.020	0.414
Time on unit ≥11 years				0.014	0.045	0.777	0.011	0.042	0.816	0.014	0.043	0.756
Nurse				0.033	0.054	0.573	0.037	0.053	0.520	0.033	0.054	0.568
Doctor				-0.059	0.063	0.405	-0.057	0.062	0.410	-0.059	0.063	0.402
Full time				0.047	0.020	0.080	0.045	0.020	0.088	0.047	0.020	0.082
Site 1 wave 2							0.056	0.019	0.041			
Site 2 wave 2							0.081	0.024	<0.001			
Site 3 wave 2							-0.035	0.011	0.029			
Site 4 wave 2							0.063	0.011	0.005			
Site 5 wave 2							0.272	0.007	<0.001			
>3 teamwork skills implemented										0.016	0.122	0.902
Coaching										-0.025	0.017	0.220
Facilitator and trained everyone										-0.008	0.021	0.716

Table G.2
Regression Results for Staff Perceptions of Communication Openness in the Labor and Delivery Unit

Result	Model 1			Model 2			Model 3			Model 4		
	Coefficient	Robust SE	p-Value	Coefficient	Robust SE	p-Value	Coefficient	Robust SE	p-Value	Coefficient	Robust SE	p-Value
Constant	0.470	0.012	<0.001	0.506	0.016	<0.001	0.536	0.009	<0.001	0.517	0.028	<0.001
Wave 2	0.031	0.032	0.395	0.028	0.031	0.427				0.023	0.057	0.707
Site 1	-0.024	0.006	0.018	-0.054	0.013	0.015	-0.090	0.011	0.001	-0.071	0.025	0.049
Site 2	0.064	0.004	<0.001	0.044	0.013	0.026	0.038	0.009	0.016	0.057	0.025	0.085
Site 4	0.073	0.006	<0.001	0.053	0.014	0.021	0.074	0.005	<0.001	0.093	0.022	0.014
Site 5	0.010	0.002	0.018	-0.019	0.017	0.316	-0.073	0.017	0.013	-0.023	0.017	0.245
Time on unit 6–10 years				0.023	0.023	0.372	0.013	0.024	0.625	0.013	0.024	0.627
Time on unit ≥11 years				0.004	0.012	0.766	-0.006	0.012	0.645	-0.004	0.014	0.779
Nurse				-0.003	0.030	0.928	-0.006	0.028	0.853	-0.008	0.029	0.809
Doctor				-0.029	0.029	0.379	-0.029	0.026	0.328	-0.031	0.026	0.307
Fulltime				-0.006	0.008	0.496	-0.009	0.009	0.420	-0.008	0.010	0.456
Site 1 wave 2							0.104	0.010	0.001			
Site 2 wave 2							-0.001	0.002	0.632			
Site 3 wave 2							-0.033	0.002	<0.001			
Site 4 wave 2							-0.057	0.008	0.003			
Site 5 wave 2							0.128	0.006	<0.001			
>3 teamwork skills implemented										-0.185	0.058	0.034
Coaching										0.105	0.012	0.001
Facilitator and trained everyone										0.160	0.008	<0.001

Table G.3
Regression Results for Staff Perceptions of Teamwork Climate in the Labor and Delivery Unit

Result	Model 1			Model 2			Model 3			Model 4		
	Coefficient	Robust SE	p-Value	Coefficient	Robust SE	p-Value	Coefficient	Robust SE	p-Value	Coefficient	Robust SE	p-Value
Constant	0.447	0.012	<0.001	0.519	0.040	<0.001	0.559	0.043	<0.001	0.542	0.044	<0.001
Wave 2	0.072	0.030	0.076	0.066	0.034	0.130				0.018	0.049	0.735
Site 1	0.147	0.006	<0.001	0.122	0.021	0.004	0.073	0.015	0.009	0.090	0.027	0.029
Site 2	0.146	0.004	<0.001	0.133	0.021	0.003	0.111	0.017	0.003	0.129	0.026	0.007
Site 4	0.336	0.006	<0.001	0.317	0.021	<0.001	0.296	0.013	<0.001	0.313	0.021	<0.001
Site 5	-0.009	0.002	0.016	-0.051	0.023	0.093	-0.100	0.025	0.015	-0.055	0.024	0.081
Time on unit 6–10 years				-0.031	0.047	0.540	-0.041	0.043	0.402	-0.041	0.043	0.403
Time on unit ≥11 years				-0.008	0.018	0.668	-0.019	0.019	0.397	-0.017	0.020	0.454
Nurse				-0.039	0.064	0.578	-0.041	0.064	0.554	-0.043	0.065	0.541
Doctor				-0.112	0.058	0.127	-0.108	0.056	0.129	-0.109	0.056	0.125
Fulltime				0.006	0.032	0.855	0.005	0.033	0.890	0.005	0.032	0.878
Site 1 wave 2							0.154	0.020	0.002			
Site 2 wave 2							0.042	0.002	<0.001			
Site 3 wave 2							-0.033	0.004	0.002			
Site 4 wave 2							0.038	0.009	0.014			
Site 5 wave 2							0.112	0.009	<0.001			
>3 teamwork skills implemented										-0.092	0.061	0.205
Coaching										0.112	0.021	0.006
Facilitator and trained everyone										0.116	0.013	0.001

Table G.4
Regression Results for Staff Quality of Work Life

Result	Model 1			Model 2			Model 3			Model 4		
	Coefficient	Robust SE	p-Value	Coefficient	Robust SE	p-Value	Coefficient	Robust SE	p-Value	Coefficient	Robust SE	p-Value
Constant	0.548	0.009	<0.001	0.539	0.047	<0.001	0.556	0.041	<0.001	0.542	0.042	<0.001
Wave 2	0.038	0.024	0.179	0.040	0.020	0.118				0.039	0.046	0.438
Site 1	0.140	0.005	<0.001	0.163	0.023	0.002	0.150	0.021	0.002	0.164	0.024	0.002
Site 2	0.143	0.003	<0.001	0.149	0.020	0.002	0.111	0.018	0.004	0.125	0.023	0.005
Site 4	0.175	0.004	<0.001	0.181	0.021	0.001	0.193	0.011	<0.001	0.207	0.020	<0.001
Site 5	0.124	0.002	<0.001	0.115	0.032	0.022	0.076	0.032	0.073	0.113	0.031	0.021
Time on unit 6–10 years				−0.050	0.030	0.172	−0.050	0.027	0.149	−0.050	0.028	0.147
Time on unit ≥11 years				−0.039	0.032	0.287	−0.042	0.031	0.246	−0.040	0.031	0.267
Nurse				−0.017	0.019	0.415	−0.015	0.018	0.452	−0.016	0.019	0.435
Doctor				−0.004	0.049	0.933	−0.006	0.049	0.909	−0.007	0.049	0.894
Full time				0.039	0.035	0.323	0.037	0.035	0.346	0.037	0.035	0.342
Site 1 wave 2							0.020	0.004	0.009			
Site 2 wave 2							0.085	0.005	<0.001			
Site 3 wave 2							−0.003	0.004	0.564			
Site 4 wave 2							−0.011	0.017	0.558			
Site 5 wave 2							0.117	0.006	<0.001			
>3 teamwork skills implemented										0.015	0.048	0.778
Coaching										−0.065	0.004	<0.001
Facilitator and trained everyone										0.031	0.017	0.141

Table G.5
Regression Results for Staff Knowledge of Teamwork

Result	Model 1			Model 2			Model 3			Model 4		
	Coefficient	Robust SE	p-Value	Coefficient	Robust SE	p-Value	Coefficient	Robust SE	p-Value	Coefficient	Robust SE	p-Value
Constant	0.628	0.009	<0.001	0.554	0.022	<0.001	0.549	0.030	<0.001	0.556	0.029	<0.001
Wave 2	0.042	0.022	0.128	0.038	0.026	0.211				0.042	0.022	0.129
Site 1	0.057	0.005	<0.001	0.099	0.006	<0.001	0.098	0.007	<0.001	0.090	0.009	0.001
Site 2	0.049	0.003	<0.001	0.073	0.013	0.006	0.110	0.006	<0.001	0.103	0.009	<0.001
Site 4	0.068	0.004	<0.001	0.081	0.006	<0.001	0.093	0.003	<0.001	0.086	0.007	<0.001
Site 5	0.065	0.002	<0.001	0.079	0.004	<0.001	0.097	0.005	<0.001	0.078	0.004	<0.001
Time on unit 6–10 years				−0.030	0.016	0.140	−0.036	0.015	0.081	−0.036	0.015	0.081
Time on unit ≥11 years				−0.017	0.038	0.680	−0.020	0.035	0.611	−0.020	0.036	0.601
Nurse				0.047	0.041	0.307	0.044	0.041	0.344	0.044	0.041	0.337
Doctor				0.101	0.043	0.081	0.101	0.043	0.079	0.101	0.043	0.079
Full time				0.024	0.012	0.117	0.024	0.012	0.114	0.024	0.012	0.117
Site 1 wave 2							0.095	0.006	<0.001			
Site 2 wave 2							−0.018	0.003	0.006			
Site 3 wave 2							0.062	0.008	0.001			
Site 4 wave 2							0.029	0.003	0.001			
Site 5 wave 2							0.003	0.002	0.126			
>3 teamwork skills implemented										−0.126	0.025	0.007
Coaching										0.113	0.003	<0.001
Facilitator and trained everyone										0.066	0.007	0.001

Bibliography

Agency for Healthcare Research and Quality, "About TeamSTEPPS," undated web page. As of January 2010:
http://teamstepps.ahrq.gov/about-2cl_3.htm

———, *Making Health Care Safer: A Critical Analysis of Patient Safety Practices*, Rockville, Md., evidence report/technology assessment 43, 2001. As of July 23, 2010:
http://archive.ahrq.gov/clinic/ptsafety/

AHRQ—*See* Agency for Healthcare Research and Quality.

Alexander, J. A., B. J. Weiner, S. M. Shortell, L. C. Baker, and M. P. Becker, "The Role of Organizational Infrastructure in Implementation of Hospitals' Quality Improvement," *Hospital Topics*, Vol. 84, No. 1, Winter 2006, pp. 11–20.

Arora, Vineet, Julia Kao, David Lovinger, Samuel C. Seiden, and David Meltzer, "Medication Discrepancies in Resident Sign-Outs and Their Potential to Harm," *Journal of General Internal Medicine*, Vol. 22, No. 12, December 2007, pp. 1751–1755.

Baker, David P., Sigrid Gustafson, Jeff Beaubien, Eduardo Salas, and Paul Barach, *Medical Teamwork and Patient Safety: The Evidence-Based Relation—Literature Review*, Rockville, Md.: Agency for Healthcare Research and Quality, 05-0053, July 2005. As of June 29, 2010:
http://www.ahrq.gov/qual/medteam/

Campion, Michael A., Gina J. Medsker, and A. Catherine Higgs, "Relations Between Work Group Characteristics and Effectiveness: Implications for Designing Effective Work Groups," *Personnel Psychology*, Vol. 46, No. 4, December 1993, pp. 823–850.

Cannon-Bowers, J. A., S. I. Tannenbaum, Eduardo Salas, C. E. Volpe, and R. Guzzo, "Defining Competencies and Establishing Team Training Requirements," in Richard A. Guzzo and Eduardo Salas, eds., *Team Effectiveness and Decision Making in Organizations*, San Francisco, Calif.: Jossey-Bass, 1995, pp. 333–380.

Cox, S., P. Wilcock, and J. Young, "Improving the Repeat Prescribing Process in a Busy General Practice: A Study Using Continuous Quality Improvement Methodology," *Quality Health Care*, Vol. 8, No. 2, June 1999, pp. 119–125.

DoD—*See* U.S. Department of Defense.

Farley, Donna O., *Evaluation Design for CAHPS Quality Improvement Demonstrations*, draft document, 2007.

Farley, Donna O., Sally C. Morton, Cheryl L. Damberg, M. Susan Ridgely, Allen Fremont, Michael D. Greenberg, Melony E. Sorbero, Stephanie S. Teleki, and Peter Mendel, *Assessment of the AHRQ Patient Safety Initiative: Moving from Research to Practice Evaluation Report II (2003–2004)*, Santa Monica, Calif.: RAND Corporation, TR-463-AHRQ, 2007. As of June 29, 2010:
http://www.rand.org/pubs/technical_reports/TR463/

Gandhi, Tejal K., Ann Louise Puopolo, Priscilla Dasse, Jennifer S. Haas, Helen R. Burstin, E. Francis Cook, and Troyen A. Brennan, "Obstacles to Collaborative Quality Improvement: The Case of Ambulatory General Medical Care," *International Journal of Quality in Health Care*, Vol. 12, No. 2, April 2000, pp. 115–123.

Glezerman, M., A. Witznitzer, H. Reuveni, and M. Mazor, "A Model of Efficient and Continuous Quality Improvement in a Clinical Setting," *International Journal for Quality in Health Care*, Vol. 11, No. 3, June 1999, pp. 227–232.

Gould, William W., "sg19: Linear Splines and Piecewise Linear Functions," *Stata Technical Bulletin 15*, September 1993, pp. 13–17.

Greene, William H., *Econometric Analysis*, 5th ed., Upper Saddle River, N.J.: Prentice Hall, 2003.

Gross, Peter A., Sheldon Greenfield, Shan Cretin, John Ferguson, Jeremy Grimshaw, Richard Grol, Niek Klazinga, Wilfried Lorenz, Gregg S. Meyer, Charles Riccobono, Stephen C. Schoenbaum, Paul Schyve, and Charles Shaw, "Optimal Methods for Guideline Implementation: Conclusions from Leeds Castle Meeting," *Medical Care*, Vol. 39, No. 8, Suppl. II, August 2001, pp. II85–II92.

Hackman, J. Richard, "The Design of Work Teams," in Jay William Lorsch, ed., *Handbook of Organizational Behavior*, Englewood Cliffs, N.J.: Prentice-Hall, 1987, pp. 315–342.

Harris, Susan, Bev Buchinski, Stefan Gryzbowski, Patti Janssen, G. W. Erle Mitchell, and Duncan Farquharson, "Induction of Labour: A Continuous Quality Improvement and Peer Review Program to Improve the Quality of Care," *Canadian Medical Association Journal*, Vol. 163, No. 9, October 31, 2000, pp. 1163–1166.

Ilgen, Daniel R., "Teams Embedded in Organizations: Some Implications," *American Psychologist*, Vol. 54, No. 2, February 1999, pp. 129–139.

Imai, Masaaki, *Kaizen (Ky'zen), the Key to Japan's Competitive Success*, New York: Random House Business Division, 1986.

Institute of Medicine, Committee on Quality of Health Care in America, *Crossing the Quality Chasm: A New Health System for the 21st Century*, Washington, D.C.: National Academy Press, 2001. As of June 29, 2010: http://www.nap.edu/catalog/10027.html

Joint Commission, "2010 National Patient Safety Goals (NPSGs): Effective July 1, 2010," c. 2010. As of July 3, 2010: http://www.jointcommission.org/PatientSafety/NationalPatientSafetyGoals/

Kachalia, Allen, Tejal K. Gandhi, Ann Louise Puopolo, Catherine Yoon, Eric J. Thomas, Richard Griffey, Troyen A. Brennan, and David M. Studdert, "Missed and Delayed Diagnoses in the Emergency Department: A Study of Closed Malpractice Claims from 4 Liability Insurers," *Annals of Emergency Medicine*, Vol. 49, No. 2, February 2007, pp. 196–205.

Kohn, Linda T., Janet Corrigan, and Molla S. Donaldson, eds., *To Err Is Human: Building a Safer Health System*, Washington, D.C.: National Academy Press, 2000. As of June 29, 2010: http://www.nap.edu/catalog/9728.html

Kuperman, G., B. James, J. Jacobsen, and R. M. Gardner, "Continuous Quality Improvement Applied to Medical Care: Experiences at LDS Hospital," *Medical Decision Making*, Vol. 11, No. 4, Suppl., October–December 1991, pp. S60–S65.

Larson, Eric B., "Measuring, Monitoring, and Reducing Medical Harm from a Systems Perspective: A Medical Director's Personal Reflections," *Academic Medicine*, Vol. 77, No. 10, October 2002, pp. 993–1000.

Laurila, J., C. G. Standertskjöld-Nordenstam, I. Suramo, E.-M. Tolppanen, Ol Tervonen, O. Korhola, and M. Brommels, "The Efficacy of a Continuous Quality Improvement (CQI) Method in a Radiological Department: Comparison with Non-CQI Control Material," *Acta Radiologica*, Vol. 42, No. 1, January 1, 2001, pp. 96–100.

Leape, Lucian L., Donald M. Berwick, and David W. Bates, "What Practices Will Most Improve Safety? Evidence-Based Medicine Meets Patient Safety," *Journal of the American Medical Association*, Vol. 288, No. 4, July 24, 2002, pp. 501–507.

Leape, Lucian L., T. A. Brennan, N. Laird, A. G. Lawthers, A. R. Localio, B. A. Barnes, L. Hebert, J. P. Newhouse, P. C. Weiler, and H. Hiatt, "The Nature of Adverse Events in Hospitalized Patients: Results of the Harvard Medical Practice Study II," *New England Journal of Medicine*, Vol. 324, No. 6, February 7, 1991, pp. 377–384.

Lindenauer, Peter K., Penelope Pekow, Kaijun Wang, Benjamin Gutierrez, and Evan M. Benjamin, "Lipid-Lowering Therapy and In-Hospital Mortality Following Major Noncardiac Surgery," *Journal of the American Medical Association*, Vol. 291, No. 17, May 5, 2004, pp. 2092–2099.

Mann, Susan, Stephen Pratt, Paul Gluck, Peter Nielsen, Daniel Risser, Penny Greenberg, Ronald Marcus, Marlene Goldman, David Shapiro, Mark Pearlman, and Benjamin Sachs, "Assessing Quality in Obstetrical Care: Development of Standardized Measures," *Joint Commission Journal on Quality and Patient Safety*, Vol. 32, No. 9, September 2006, pp. 497–505.

McGrath, Joseph Edward, *Groups: Interaction and Performance*, Englewood Cliffs, N.J.: Prentice-Hall, 1984.

Messina, Jeanette, "Development and Implementation of a Perioperative Assistant Training Program," *Association of Operating Room Nurses*, Vol. 66, No. 5, November 1997, pp. 890–904.

Miles, Matthew B., and A. M. Huberman, *Qualitative Data Analysis: An Expanded Sourcebook*, 2nd ed., Thousand Oaks, Calif.: Sage Publications, 1994.

Morey, John C., and Mary Salisbury, "Introducing Teamwork Training into Healthcare Organizations: Implementation Issues and Solutions," *Human Factors and Ergonomics Society Annual Meeting Proceedings*, Vol. 46, Training, 2002, pp. 2069–2073.

Morey, John C., Robert Simon, Gregory D. Jay, and Matthew M. Rice, "A Transition from Aviation Crew Resource Management to Hospital Emergency Departments: The MedTeams Story," *Proceedings of the 12th International Symposium on Aviation Psychology*, 2002, pp. 826–832.

Morey, John C., Robert Simon, Gregory D. Jay, Robert L. Wears, Mary Salisbury, Kimberly A. Dukes, and Scott D. Berns, "Error Reduction and Performance Improvement in the Emergency Department Through Formal Teamwork Training: Evaluation Results of the MedTeams Project," *Health Services Research*, Vol. 37, No. 6, December 2002, pp. 1553–1581.

National Quality Forum, *Safe Practices for Better Healthcare, A Consensus Report*, Washington, D.C., 2003.

———, *Safe Practices for Better Healthcare, 2006 Update: A Consensus Report*, Washington, D.C., 2007.

———, *Safe Practices for Better Healthcare, 2009 Update: A Consensus Report*, Washington, D.C., 2009.

Nielsen, Peter E., Marlene B. Goldman, Susan Mann, David E. Shapiro, Ronald G. Marcus, Stephen D. Pratt, Penny Greenberg, Patricia McNamee, Mary Salisbury, David J. Birnbach, Paul A. Gluck, Mark D. Pearlman, Heidi King, David N. Tornberg, and Benjamin P. Sachs, "Effects of Teamwork Training on Adverse Outcomes and Process of Care in Labor and Delivery: A Randomized Controlled Trial," *Obstetrical and Gynecological Survey*, Vol. 62, No. 5, May 2007, pp. 294–295.

NQF—*See* National Quality Forum.

O'Neil, Harold F. Jr., Gregory K. W. K. Chung, and Richard S. Brown, "Use of Networked Simulations as a Context to Measure Team Competencies," in Harold F. O'Neil Jr., ed., *Workforce Readiness: Competencies and Assessment*, Mahwah, N.J.: Lawrence Erlbaum Associates, 1997, pp. 411–452.

Panis, Constantijn, "sg24: The Piecewise Linear Spline Transformation," *Stata Technical Bulletin 18*, March 1994, pp. 27–29.

Petersen, Laura A., Troyen A. Brennan, Anne C. O'Neil, E. Francis Cook, and Thomas H. Lee, "Does Housestaff Discontinuity of Care Increase the Risk for Preventable Adverse Events?" *Annals of Internal Medicine*, Vol. 121, No. 11, December 1, 1994, pp. 866–872.

Pronovost, Peter J., and Christine G. Holzmueller, "Partnering for Quality," *Journal of Critical Care*, Vol. 19, No. 3, September 2004, pp. 121–129.

Ryan, Gery W., and H. Russell Bernard, "Data Management and Analysis Methods," in Norman K. Denzin and Yvonna S. Lincoln, eds., *Handbook of Qualitative Research*, 2nd ed., Thousand Oaks, Calif.: Sage Publications, 2000, pp. 769–802.

Rycroft-Malone, J., A. Kitson, G. Harvey, B. McCormack, K. Seers, A. Titchen, and C. Estabrooks, "Ingredients for Change: Revisiting a Conceptual Framework," *Quality and Safety in Health Care*, Vol. 11, No. 2, 2002, pp. 174–180.

Salas, E., L. Rhodenizer, and C. A. Bowers, "The Design and Delivery of Crew Resource Management Training: Exploiting Available Resources," *Human Factors*, Vol. 42, No. 3, 2000, pp. 490–511.

Schwab, R. A., S. M. DelSorbo, M. R. Cunningham, K. Craven, and W. A. Watson, "Using Statistical Process Control to Demonstrate the Effect of Operational Interventions on Quality Indicators in the Emergency Department," *Journal of Healthcare Quality*, Vol. 21, No. 4, July–August 1999, pp. 38–41.

Sexton, J. B., E. J. Thomas, R. L. Helmreich, T. B. Neilands, K. Rowan, K. Vella, J. Boyden, and P. R. Roberts, *Frontline Assessments of Healthcare Culture: Safety Attitudes Questionnaire Norms and Psychometric Properties*, Houston, Texas: University of Texas Center of Excellence for Patient Safety Research and Practice, technical report 04-01, 2004.

Silverman, Myrna, Edmund M. Ricci, and Margaret J. Gunter, "Strategies for Increasing the Rigor of Qualitative Methods in Evaluation of Health Care Programs," *Evaluation Review*, Vol. 14, No. 1, 1990, pp. 57–74.

Solberg, Leif I., Milo L. Brekke, Thomas E. Kottke, and Robert P. Steel, "Continuous Quality Improvement in Primary Care: What's Happening?" *Medical Care*, Vol. 36, No. 5, May 1998, pp. 625–635.

Sorbero, Melony E., Donna O. Farley, Soeren Mattke, and Susan L. Lovejoy, *Outcome Measures for Effective Teamwork in Inpatient Care: Final Report*, Santa Monica, Calif.: RAND Corporation, TR-462-AHRQ, 2008. As of July 1, 2010:
http://www.rand.org/pubs/technical_reports/TR462/

Sorra, Joann, and Veronica F. Nieva, *Hospital Survey on Patient Safety Culture*, Rockville, Md.: Agency for Healthcare Research and Quality, publication 04-0041, September 2004. As of July 1, 2010:
http://permanent.access.gpo.gov/lps83504/hospcult.pdf

Stata Corporation, *Stata 8: Statistics, Graphics, Data Management*, College Station, Texas, 2003.

Stevens, Michael J., and Michael A. Campion, "The Knowledge, Skill, and Ability Requirements for Teamwork: Implications for Human Resource Management," *Journal of Management*, Vol. 20, No. 2, 1994, pp. 503–530.

Strauss, Anselm L., and Juliet M. Corbin, *Basics of Qualitative Research: Techniques and Procedures for Developing Grounded Theory*, 2nd ed., Thousand Oaks, Calif.: Sage Publications, 1998.

Taylor, S. L., S. Ridgely, M. D. Greenberg, M. E. Sorbero, S. S. Teleki, C. L., Damberg, and D. O. Farley, "Experiences of AHRQ-Funded Projects That Implemented Practices for Safer Patient Care," *Health Services Research*, Vol. 44, No. 2, Part II, April 2009, pp. 665–683.

U.S. Department of Defense, *TeamSTEPPS Pocket Guide*, Falls Church, Va.: TRICARE Management Activity, 2005.